Sayed Abdulrazek
Sharifa Alaraimi
Aya Youssef

The Medical Interpreter bookPart 1

Sayed Abdulrazek
Sharifa Alaraimi
Aya Youssef

The Medical Interpreter bookPart 1

Introduction, English-Arabic Glossary, Scenarios& Games

Noor Publishing

Imprint

Any brand names and product names mentioned in this book are subject to trademark, brand or patent protection and are trademarks or registered trademarks of their respective holders. The use of brand names, product names, common names, trade names, product descriptions etc. even without a particular marking in this work is in no way to be construed to mean that such names may be regarded as unrestricted in respect of trademark and brand protection legislation and could thus be used by anyone.

Cover image: www.ingimage.com

Publisher:
Noor Publishing
is a trademark of
Dodo Books Indian Ocean Ltd. and OmniScriptum S.R.L publishing group

120 High Road, East Finchley, London, N2 9ED, United Kingdom
Str. Armeneasca 28/1, office 1, Chisinau MD-2012, Republic of Moldova, Europe
Printed at: see last page
ISBN: 978-620-5-63786-9

PART 1

The Medical Interpreter Book

Introduction | English –Arabic Glossary | Scenarios & Games

El-Sayed Abdulrazek

Maysaa Khattab | Sharifa Alaraimi | Aya Youssef Ismail

كتاب المترجم الطبي الشفوي (التتابعي)

مقدمة عن تاريخ الترجمة | مسرد المصطلحات ثنائي اللغة "عربي – انجليزي" | سيناريوهات ترجمة وألعاب تفاعلية

السيد عبد الرازق

ميساء خطاب | شريفة العَرِيمِي | آية يوسف إسماعيل

Table of Contents

Section 1

My book is uniquely different from any other book covering the same topic. Existing books on medical interpretation focus only on the roles and responsibilities of interpreters, and mentioning the techniques used for effective interpretation. Still other medical interpretation books have poor coverage of bilingual medical terminology, not including common dialect differences; leading to medical interpreters having to do their own research, which leads to higher rates of mistakes or misunderstandings occurring. This is unacceptable in any field, let alone in a medical interpretation, where a patient's health and well-being are at stake.

My book encompasses both components of this skillset, incorporating the rules and regulations as well as an introduction to human anatomy and medical terminology in both languages.
It includes:
- Bilingual terminology for every term used in medical interpretation
- 50+ medical terminologies of symptoms for each specialty
- 60+ medical terminologies of diseases for each specialty
- 20+ medical terminologies of investigations/tests for each specialty
- 30+ medical terminologies of surgical interventions for each specialty
- More than 40 pages of the Latin prefixes and suffixes used to construct all medical terminology, including their interpretation into English and Arabic and example for each.
- An interactive part! Have fun solving puzzles and crosswords that help the novice interpreter memorize all the terminology.
- Real life scenarios for the absolute novice to practice interpreting

The chapters of my book are divided into different medical sciences found in a hospital setting and some will be sub-divided even further for ease of use. For example: Orthopedics chapter is subdivided into Upper and Lower limbs and further sub-divided into individual joints. They include bilingual terminology for the anatomy, symptoms, investigations, diseases and disorders, as well as treatments, both conservative and surgical.

Although this is book is comprehensive, it does not cover ALL hospital departments and I intend to continue in a second book.

Accuracy-wise the Medical terminology part has been reviewed by specialist doctor from worldwide for each specialty. Who speaks English and other native languages 13 languages (English, Arabic, Danish, French, German, Hindi, Korean, Malayalam, Norwegian, Spanish, Swedish, Tamil, Telugu, Urdu)

El-Sayed Abdelrazek is well-trained Medical & Community Arabic – English Interpreter & HIPAA compliant with over 17 years of experience. Currently working in the United Arab Emirates as an onsite medical interpreter, and also provide remote interpreting OPI and VRI for clients in the U.S., U.K. and Canada for 2000 hours.

استهلال Preface

إهداء

- إلى روح أبي وجدتي عزيزة...

اهدي هذا الكتاب والاستفادة منه إلى روح والدي الحاج/ عبد الرازق السيد الذي جاور ربه ورحل عن الدنيا فجأة بدون أي حسبان، وجدتي التي ترملت في عُمر صغير وصبرت ورضيت بقضاء الله وكدت في حياتها لتربية أبنائها الصغار.

- وإلى عائلتي الصغيرة...

زوجتي وأولادي جنى ومروان وعمر

على كل فرد رسم حلم وخطة في حياته، لجعلها ملينة بالتحديات وذات هدف، وعليه أن يعمل ويسعى ويحاول ويجتهد لتحقيق هذا الحلم، وحتى لو أخبروك الناس من حولك بأنه صعب المنال.

أحبكم كثيرا

- وإلى كل انسان عربي من الخليج للمحيط لديه الشغف للعمل في مجال الترجمة الطبية الشفوية...

أتمنى أن يكون كتابي بمثابة بذرة تنير بها دروب حياتكم العملية، والتعرف على أهمية مساهمتكم السامية في مجال الرعاية الصحية.

أخيرًا وليس آخرًا

- إلى أكاديمية ابن سينا ود. ميسم مجدي (المدير التنفيذي)...

اعتبر ابن سينا نقطة تحول هامة في حياتي، من خلال اتاحة فرصة تعلم أساسيات الترجمة الطبية بشكل احترافي عن طريق دوراتهم المكثفة في الترجمة الطبية، ومن ثم التحول الجذري في مساري المهني.

ممتن لكل أفراد عائلة ابن سينا

مقدمة Introduction

ميزنا الخالق سبحانه وتعالى نحن البشر بلغات وألسنة مختلفة التي نستخدمها للتعبير عن احتياجتنا وللتواصل مع الآخرين. والتعبير عن مشاعرنا المتضاربة من حزن، فرح، آلام. اللغة ليست مجرد كلمات بل هي أشمل وأعمق، حيث تعبر اللغة عن ثقافات وحضارات وقيم وأخلاق شعوب وقبائل. وحتى نتمكن من استيعاب وفهم لغة بعينها نحتاج لدراسة وفهم كل ما يدور حول الأنسان المتحدث لهذه اللغة من خلفية ثقافية، دين، تاريخ وموروثات مجتمعية، عادات وتقاليد. وكيفية تعبيره عن مشاعره بالكلمات والعبارات المختلفة وطريقة تعبير لغة الجسد ونبرة الصوت في هذه اللغة، مثالا حيث بعض المجتمعات تعتبر نبرة الصوت المرتفعة تعبيرا عن الحماس والفرح، وشعوب أخرى تعبر عن الغضب...

تعلم لغات الشعوب يساعد الناس على التواصل وفهم بعضهم بعضا والتعاون على خير الإنسانية جمعاء كما قال الله تعالى في القرآن الكريم يَا أَيُّهَا النَّاسُ إِنَّا خَلَقْنَاكُم مِّن ذَكَرٍ وَأُنثَىٰ وَجَعَلْنَاكُمْ شُعُوبًا وَقَبَائِلَ لِتَعَارَفُوا ۚ إِنَّ أَكْرَمَكُمْ عِندَ اللَّهِ أَتْقَاكُمْ ۚ إِنَّ اللَّهَ عَلِيمٌ خَبِيرٌ (13)

لذا اعتبر وظيفة الترجمة مهنة سامية، لتقريب الناس ومساعدتهم على فهم واستيعاب الاختلافات البينية في شكل حضاري. فنحن كمترجمين لسنا قواميس متنقلة أو انسان آلي للترجمة، لكن الدور المنوط هو ترجمة أفكار، كلمات، مشاعر، لغة جسد، نبرة صوت، حياة انسان كاملة لمساعدة الناس على فهم بعض بشكل أفضل.

لذا فكرت في فكرة الكتاب عن الترجمة الشفوية في مجال الرعاية الصحية، حيث يختلف عن باقي الكتب في هذا السياق حيث هنا جمعت كل ما يحتاجه المترجم بشكل شامل، عن طريق طرح الكتاب في ثلاثة أقسام مهمة لكل مترجم طبي عربي – اتجليزي معاصر

القسم الأول:

يقوم بطرح وسرد تاريخ الترجمة الشفوية، والفرق بين الترجمة التحريرية والشفوية، الأدوار الأربعة للمترجم الشفوي الذي من خلالها يستطيع أن يترجم بشكل احترافي ومتى يتنقل بين الأربعة أدوار باحترافية على حسب الموقف، قواعد الترجمة الطبية التي يجب علينا الالتزام بها HIPAA Complaint ، (The Health Insurance Portability and Accountability Act)

(قاعدة حفظ الخصوصيات التابعة لقانون إخضاع التأمين الصحي لقابلية النقل والمحاسبة)

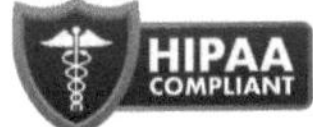

والتعرف على أنواع الترجمة الشفوية المختلفة، أخلاقيات الترجمة الطبية

القسم الثاني:

يتضمن ترجمة كل البادءات واللاحقات الطبية(prefixes and suffixes) بشكل مبسط مع أمثلتها في شكل مصطلحات طبية، وأيضا يتضمن 15 تخصص من مجالات الطب وسرد المصطلحات باللغتين العربية والأنجليزية، من عرض الجزء التشريحي لهذا التخصص، أعراض المرض، الأمراض، الفحوصات المطلوبة، العلاجات المتوفرة، الإجراءات الطبية/العمليات الجراحية، المضاعفات في حالة عدم البدء في العلاج أو في فترة التشافي بعد الجراحة أو أثناء العمليات لكل تخصص على حدا على سبيل المثال لا الحصر تخصص طب الأسرة، العظام، العمود الفقري،.....

القسم الثالث:

يتضمن جزء تفاعلي من سيناريوهات حقيقية بين المريض والطبيب في عيادات مختلفة مع الترجمة من وإلى اللغتين العربية والانجليزية، ومن ثم ترك مجال لبعض السيناريوهات بدون ترجمة للتدريب عليها،

وأيضا يتضمن الجزء الثالث أسئلة وفوازير وكلمات متقاطعة عن المصطلحات الطبية والأمراض بشكل شيق وتفاعلي للتدريب أتمنى أن يفي هذا الكتاب بالغرض المنوط منه لتلبية ومساعدة كل مترجم طبي عربي انجليزي في مجال عمله وتعزيز وفهم مدى أهمية الدور الحيوي الذي يقوم به في مجال الرعاية الصحية، والتأكيد على أن غياب المترجم في المنظومة الصحية يسبب خلل في التواصل بين المريض ومقدمي الرعاية الصحية والذي يترتب عليه أخطاء جسيمة في التشخيصات الطبية والعلاجات المترتبة على ذلك والتي تؤثر على صحة وحياة المريض.

- عذرا مسبقا عن أي أخطاء غير مقصودة في الكتاب-

Acknowledgment

Immeasurable appreciation and deepest gratitude are extended to the following physicians for their help and support of our endeavor through medical review of the terminology in English and Arabic and who did the needful amendments and shared their professional experience.

#	Physician name	Specialty	Spoken languages
1	Dr. Nikhil Dinakar Thada MBBS, DLO, DNB	ENT	English
2	Dr. Hachem Jammal	ENT	English & Arabic
3	Dr. Seif Sawalha MBBS, MRCS, FRCS, CCT	Elbow Orthopedic Surgery	English & Arabic
4	Dr. Borja Merry Del Val MBBS, FEBOT, MRCS	Orthopedic Surgery	English & Spanish
5	Dr. Sami Hassan BMedSci, MBChB, MRCS , FRCS	Hand Surgery	Urdu & English
6	Dr. Musab Abdallah MBBS, FRCS	Orthopedic Surgery	English & Arabic
7	Dr. Martin Falken Wetterhall MBBS, M.D.	Orthopedic Spinal Surgery	English & Swedish
8	Dr. Kiyoung Choi Consultant M.D. FABMISS	Neurological Surgery	English & Korean
9	Dr. Waleed Hekal MBBCh, MSc (Orth), MD (Orth), FRCS (Eng), FRCS (Glasg), FRCSI, FRCS [Tr&Orth]	Spine Surgery	English & Arabic
10	Dr. Zahid Raza MBChB, MD, FRCSEd	Vascular Surgery	Urdu & English
11	Dr. John Paul MBBS Bsc, FRCP, MD (Res)	Cardiology	English, French & German
12	Dr. Rami Harb	Cardiology	English & Arabic
13	Dr. Sheik Ryaz Yaseen M.D.	Neurology	English, Norwegian, Swedish, Danish, Tamil
14	Dr. Leanne Brown DClinPsyh, QiCN	Clinical Neuropsychology	English
15	Dr. Zaki Abou Zahr FACR, RhMSUS, RMSK, CCD	Rheumatology	English & Arabic
16	Dr. Favas Thaivalappil MRCP, FRCP, CCT, Post-CCT Fellowship	Pulmonology & Sleep Medicine	English, Malayalam & Hindi
17	Dr. Nauman Chaudhry MRCP, FRCP, CCT	Pulmonology & Sleep Medicine	English, Urdu, Telugu
18	Dr Jassem Abdou	Respiratory and Sleep medicine-Pulmonologist	English & Arabic
19	Dr. Hudhaifa Almukhtar FRCS, FACS	General Surgeon	English & Arabic
20	Dr. Sagar Jujjavarapu MBBS, MRCP	Nephrology	English & Tamil
21	Dr. Laith Al-Rubaiy	Gastroenterology & Hepatology	English & Arabic

About Assistant Authors

This book would not have been possible without the assistance of these interpreters and their willingness to share their professional experience to help trainees and those interested in this field, to open a new road of opportunities to becoming medical interpreters.

#	Interpreter	Country	Expertise
1	Maysaa Khattab	State of Palestine	15 years in healthcare
2	Sharifa Alaraimi	Oman & UK	11 years in healthcare
3	Aya Ismail Yousef	State of Palestine	7 years in healthcare

Assisted and contributed in Section/Chapter	Assistant Author
• Neurology & Neuropsychology • Crossword games	Sharifa Alaraimi
• Medical prefixes and suffixes (N-Z) • Anatomy and Physiology • Shoulder • Elbow	Aya Ismail Yousef
• Gastroenterology • Urology & Gynecology • Surgery • Vascular • Nephrology	Maysaa Khattab

The History of Language Interpretation and translation

The birth of translation and interpretation is known to date back to earlier than 300 B.C. in Ancient Egypt. There are no confirmed evidence of translation or interpretation activities prior to the Ancient Egyptian dealings with the Dynasty of Nubia, Ancient Greece and the Roman Empire. The first record of interpreting activity were in the form of Egyptian low-relief sculptures found in a prince's tomb, that made reference to an interpreter supervisor. Therefore, scholars agree that the history of interpretation and translation began in Egypt, since it is there that civilization, in its own sense was born and constructed: one of the earliest forms of writing was born there, with which the history of civilized society began.

The earliest known graphic depiction of an interpreter at work

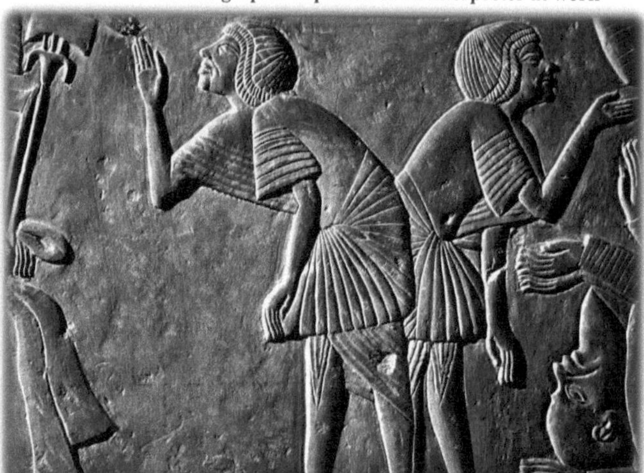

The tomb of Haremhab (or Horemhab) at Saqqara, ancient Memphis, just outside Cairo. It dates from about 1330 BCE.

How did we understand the Ancient Egyptian hieroglyphs and its civilization?

For centuries, life in ancient Egypt was a mystery, until the discovery of "the Rosetta Stone حجر رشيد", by a Frenchman named Bouchard in August 1799. In 1814, the Englishman Thomas Young, and later in 1821-22, the Frenchman Jean-François Champollion; interpreted and deciphered the languages engraved on the stone: Hieroglyphics, Demotic and Ancient Greek - اللغة المصرية القديمة الهيروغليفية المصرية، و الهيراطيقية (الديموطقية)، و اليونانية القديمة(الإغريقية)

The inscriptions, apparently composed by the priests of Memphis, summarize benefactions conferred by Ptolemy V Epiphanes (205–180 BCE) and were written in the ninth year of his reign in commemoration of his accession to the throne.

Interpreters continued to be employed throughout the Middle Ages. Monks of many different nationalities translated Biblical texts in monasteries;

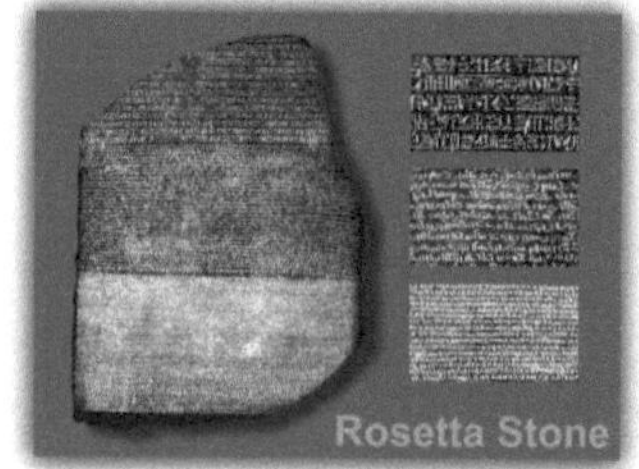

preachers of foreign lands interpreted in councils, as well as some individuals interpreted/translated on business expeditions, military incursions and diplomatic meetings.

During the Age of Discovery (1400s-1600s), the discovery of new trade routes opened up the European nations to many different, new languages, which greatly changed the way we see interpretation today. For example, Christopher Columbus, in 1492, thought that he could sail West across the Atlantic, to India. He accidentally led the Spanish to the discovery of the Americas, although he also led to inadvertantly naming the indigenous people 'Indians'. In this, his first voyage, he noted that his Arabic and Hebrew-speaking interpreters were not very helpful in communicating with the indigenous peoples. After this voyage, he decided to capture some Native Americans and teach them Spanish so they could help him as interpreters on his next expedition.

How did medical interpretation become essential in healthcare industry in US?
Implications of Language Barriers for Healthcare: A Systematic Review

Hilal Al Shamsi,[1,*] Abdullah G. Almutairi,[2] Sulaiman Al Mashrafi,[3] and Talib Al Kalbani[4]

Many patients with limited English proficiency experienced adverse health events that resulted in detectable physical harm (49.1% of patients) or moderate temporary harm (46.8%) or experienced some failure in communication with medical providers (52.4%).5 Patients with limited English language proficiency are also likely to miss medical appointments and have difficulties arranging appointments due to the language barrier. Therefore, these patients have a poor level of satisfaction with their healthcare.

To increase patient satisfaction with healthcare, it is necessary to provide interpreter services. Two studies pointed out that medical providers needed interpreter services for 43.2% of their patients, and 21–76% of medical providers stated they had poor access to these services. Moreover, 70.7% of limited English proficiency patients (LEPPs) reported limited availability of interpreter services, and 26.4% reported that there were no interpreters in their healthcare institutions.

Translating from one language to another is a tricky business, and when it comes to interpreting between a doctor and a patient, the stakes are even higher. In medical situations, sometimes doctors and their clinical teams turn to a patients' family members for help with interpreting, but that can be problematic as well. It must be communicated through a well-trained professional medical interpreter to avoid any malpractice and/or misdiagnosis that may lead to serious impacts on a patient's health.

Medical Tragedy: The Case Of Willie Ramirez 18-year old baseball player

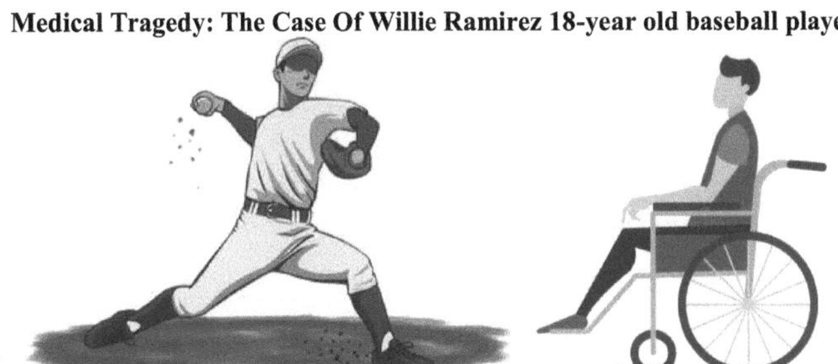

Expressive images of Medical Tragedy: The Case Of Willie Ramirez 18-year old baseball player

I am going to narrate the tale of a lovely 18-year old Cuban named Willie Ramirez, who used to have fun and play his favorite sports game, baseball, with his friends. One day Ramirez felt unwell, gradually getting worse until he passed out. He was brought into a South Florida emergency room, and when the doctors asked his family what happened to him, and to get his medical history so that they can help him and treat him accordingly. Unfortunately, his mother only spoke Spanish, and his girlfriends' mother only spoke a little English but she tried to convey that Willie was 'INTOXICADO'. The medical team misinterpreted the term as 'intoxicated' as through a drug overdose, and instructed the treatment accordingly. However, the word 'INTOXICADO', in Spanish, means sickness due to something you took orally like a food or drink. His family thought that he got sick from fast food he had eaten earlier that day. A couple of days later, the doctors found out that the actual diagnosis was cerebral hemorrhage with brain stem compression, that was almost too late to treat even with emergency surgery. The poor young man had become quadriplegic, i.e. the paralysis of all four limbs.

Now the hospital is liable for a settlement of approximately 71 million dollars to pay for Willie's care for the rest of his life according to a 2002 report from the US Office of Management and Budget.

US Regulation has mandated the requirement to provide Interpreters for all non-English speaking patients
The law is title six of the Civil Rights Act of 1964 section 157 of the Patient Protection and Affordable Care Act and the Americans with Disabilities Act have been written to improve communication with patients of limited English proficiency.

What does this mean in practical terms?

All healthcare providers receiving federal financial assistance are now required by law to provide interpreters for all non-english speaking patients.

Interpretation VS Translation

TRANSLATORS vs INTERPRETERS

While both translators and interpreters transfer meaning between languages, there's a big difference between what they do and the skills they possess. This simple infographic will help you determine which type you need.

WRITE
It's simple:
translators write...

SPEAK
...and interpreters speak.

DELAYED
Your final translation product will take days or longer

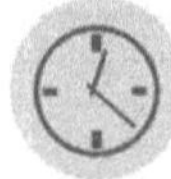

REAL-TIME
The final product is delivered instantly

TARGET LANGUAGE
Translators don't have to be conversationally fluent in their source language but must be in the target language

BOTH LANGUAGES
It's essential that interpreters are native or near native in both langauges

DICTIONARIES
Translators rely on numerous industry-specific resources

ON-THE-SPOT
When on the job, interpreters do not have consult dictionaries, glossaries, etc.

EXAMPLE: LEGAL CONTRACT
A contract is a common example of a translation product

EXAMPLE: BUSINESS MEETING
Conducting a meeting? You will need an interpreter!

Translation: الترجمة التحريرية (المكتوبة)

Works with the written language from one language to another. Converting words from a source language to a target language. It must preserving the register and meaning of the source language content.

Interpretation: الترجمة الشفوية (المنطوقة/المحكية)

Works with the spoken language or with Sign Language, converting oral phrases, ideas and idioms from a source language to a target language almost instantly, while preserving the register and meaning of the source language content.

In short, translation and interpretation bridge the language gap between people in two different countries and cultures.

*Some terminology you need to be familiar with when you work in interpretation

	Job role	باللغة العربية	Job title	باللغة العربية
1	Translation	ترجمة تحريرية (نصية/مكتوبة)	Translator	مترجم تحريري "مترجم النصوص"
2	Interpretation	ترجمة شفوية (منطوقة/محكية)	Interpreter	ترجمان "مترجم شفوي" "مترجم اللغة المحكية"
3	Arabic Sign Language (ArSL)	لغة الإشارة العربية		Arabic sign language (ArSL) is a full natural language that is used by the deaf in Arab countries to communicate in their community. Unfamiliarity with this language increases the isolation of deaf people from society. This language has a different structure, word order, and lexicon than Arabic.
4	**LEP** "Limited Englishh Proficient"	المريض/العميل الفرد الذي يجيد اللغة الإنجليزية بشكل محدود		*The Department of Justice defines **LEP** as follows: If these individuals have a limited ability to read, write, speak, or understand English, they are limited English proficient, or "**LEP**."
5	Provider	الطبيب/مقدم الخدمة الشخص الذي يجيد اللغة الإنجليزية بطلاقة		A healthcare provider is a person or entity that provides medical care or treatment. Healthcare providers include doctors, nurse practitioners, midwives, radiologists, labs, hospitals, urgent care clinics, medical supply companies, and other professionals, facilities, and businesses that provide such services.
6	Source language	اللغة المصدر (اللغة الأصلية)		is the language being translated from.
7	Target language	اللغة المستهدفة		is the language being translated into.

*For example, if I interpret from Japanese to English, then **my source language** is Japanese and **my target language** is English.
*Also, if I work from **source** documents in Japanese and translate them into **target** documents in English.
What is Interpretation?

Interpreting services function as a verbal form of translation that is facilitated by a professional interpreter, or a team of interpreters. Interpretation services are used to translate speeches, presentations, conversations, and other spoken languages into the native or preferred language of a given audience.

Interpretation is considered as the art of transforming a message from one language to another, either through speaking or signing. Unlike translation, which involves written communication, interpretation is done verbally or through sign language. This crucial distinction between the two is what sets them apart.

By providing interpreting services to your audience, you can communicate across language barriers essentially in real-time, expediting the speed at which information can be delivered while allowing them to benefit from the context in which the speech is provided. Members of a presentation audience, for example, can view visual aids or slideshows as an interpreter provides insights and explanations for those slides.

Types of interpretation:

	Type of interpretation	نوع الترجمة
1	Consecutive Interpretation	ترجمة تتابعية
2	Simultaneous Interpretation	ترجمة فورية متزامنة
3	Whispered Interpretation (Chuchotage)	ترجمة همسية
4	Relay Interpretation	ترجمة مرحلية
5	Liaison Interpretation (dialogue interpretation)	ترجمة الربط
6	Sight Interpretation	ترجمة منظورة
7	Escort or Travel Interpretation	ترجمة مرافق السفر والسياحة
	Remote Interpretation	**ترجمة عن بعد**
8	Over-the-phone Interpreting (OPI)	الترجمة الفورية عبر الهاتف
9	Video Remote Interpreting (VRI)	الترجمة الفورية عبر الفيديو

1. Consecutive Interpreting

This type of interpretation requires the interpreter to wait for the speaker to finish their speech or statement before proceeding to deliver that same message in the target language. Since the interpreter has to wait for the speaker to finish talking, they usually take notes to remember what's being said and later use them to deliver the interpretation.

With consecutive interpretation, speakers will talk for up to five minutes or longer before taking a break to allow interpretation to occur. Consecutive interpreting allows for a back-and-forth between multiple parties, which is why it's a popular approach used in medical, legal proceedings and business meetings.

Interpreters taking on a consecutive interpretation assignment must have a strong memory and note-taking skills to keep information organized over minutes-long stretches of speech. Accuracy in interpreting is critical even when the interpreter must convey the contents of a long speech, which is why it's crucial to enlist the help of a certified, experienced interpreting expert.

2. Simultaneous Interpreting

Unlike consecutive interpretation, simultaneous interpretation does not wait for a break in a speech to translate into the target language. Instead, simultaneous interpreting takes place over the speech as it's taking place, usually with a delay of 30 seconds or less.

This type of interpretation places a lot of pressure on the interpreter, who must be able to translate from one language into the next and convey that content to an audience, while also listening to a real-time speech as it progresses and comprehending how it should be interpreted.

Simultaneous interpretation is also intended to provide an exact conversion of speech from one language into another, rather than paraphrasing. In some cases, the audience receiving this interpretation will wear headphones so they can hear the interpretation without interference from surrounding noise, while also paying attention to any presentation taking place.

Simultaneous interpreting is popular at big meetings or gatherings where a large audience must be engaged in multiple languages. The United Nations is a popular example of this type of interpreting since many members of the assembly wear headphones to hear interpretations into the language of their choice.

It's also widely used in smaller conferences, board meetings of large multinationals, international court hearings, etc.

*Due to the workload of simultaneous interpreting, interpreters will sometimes work in teams of two or more to facilitate a smooth performance. These teams can also function at the live event itself or from a remote location.

3. Whisper Interpreting

This type of interpreting is similar to simultaneous interpretation, with one key difference: Instead of using microphones and headsets to communicate with intended audience members, the interpreter will sit with an individual or group of people needing interpretive services, and the interpreter will whisper in their preferred language to facilitate communication across language barriers. Protranslating also uses whisper sound technology to speak to an audience within close range of the speaker.

Whisper interpreting is best used with a small group of people who need interpretation, especially when the facility lacks the technology required to provide headset-based interpretive services. Whisper interpreting can also be used in business or diplomatic meetings where individuals require the help of an interpreter.

4. Relay interpreting /indirect interpreting.

During relay interpreting, the interpreter listens to the source language speaker and renders the message into a language common to all the other interpreters. These other interpreters then render the message to their target language groups.

Relay interpreting is one of the many forms of interpreting services. Its seamless execution disguises its use particularly in large conferences.

When relay interpreting it used, an interpreter listens to the speaker and translates the message into a language known by the rest of the interpreting team, who then interpret the message they have received into the languages spoken by each of their target groups.

5. Liaison interpreting

While some authors see liaison interpreting as a type of consecutive interpreting, both types have their distinguishing characteristics. The two most significant aspects of liaison interpreting, in this regard, are that it does not tend to require note-taking and that it is performed in a two-way manner. As such, liaison interpreting does not require such a thorough preparation from the professional compared to other types of interpreting. However, excellent language proficiency in both working languages is essential. The aim is to guarantee spontaneous and fluent communication, adapted to the situation, in which the most appropriate vocabulary is employed. **Liaison,** also known as **bilateral or accompanying interpreting** is used in very small debate groups, commercial and touristic visits, exhibition and factory visits, tours of plants and other facilities, training courses and more.

6. Sight interpretation

This is the interpretation of a written text received by the translator, usually without any time for preparation. Such interpreting services are usually delivered by a certified translator at a notary's office or in a courtroom, when an interested party must be made familiar with the contents of a document presented in a foreign language.

Sight interpretation requires excellent language skills, a good memory, quick thinking, resistance to stress, and good powers of attention and concentration on the part of the interpreter. The greatest challenge for the interpreter is the lack of familiarity with the contents and the context of the entire document while being expected to read and translate the required fragments. To make the translation correct, coherent and fluent, the translator must take in as much of the text as possible and be able to translate it into the target language immediately.

7. Escort/Travel Interpreting

Another type of consecutive interpretation, escort interpretation (also known as travel interpretation) is very similar to liaison interpretation. The difference is that these interpreter types are expected to accompany the client to a range of venues. That could include attending business dinners and business trips, sightseeing while overseas, attending cultural events and so forth.

From the interpreter's perspective, this can be an exciting way to see more of the world while also being paid to do so!

For individuals or select groups requiring dedicated interpretation throughout a foreign visit or other events, escort/travel interpretation can provide custom, personal interpreting services in any location.

These interpreters travel with individuals or small groups wherever they go on a business or diplomatic trip, providing interpretive services in a range of settings. In addition to business meetings and presentations, these interpreters can also assist clients at restaurants, retail shops, or any other location these individuals might travel. In this way, escort interpreters can also function as cultural guides that help clients navigate the complexities and cultural considerations of traveling in another country.

8. Over-the-phone Interpreting OPI

Over-the-phone interpretation **(OPI)** is a type of interpretation that allows you to communicate with people who speak different languages over the phone. OPI is a great option for businesses that need to communicate with international clients or customers, as it provides a fast and convenient way to connect with people from all over the world.

OPI works by having the interpreter listen to your conversation over the phone, and then translate it into the desired language.

10. Video remote interpretation (VRI)

This requires the use of videoconferencing technology, equipment, and an internet connection with sufficient bandwidth to provide the services of a qualified interpreter, usually located at a call center, to people at a different location.

Video remote interpretation **(VRI)** is a type of interpretation that allows you to communicate with people who speak different languages through video conferencing. VRI is a great option for businesses that need to have face-to-face communication with international clients or customers.

VRI works by placing the interpreter in front of a camera, so they can see both you and the person you are speaking to. This allows for more accurate translations, as the interpreter can see the facial expressions and body language of both parties.

HIPAA Regulations

The Health Insurance Portability and Accountability Act

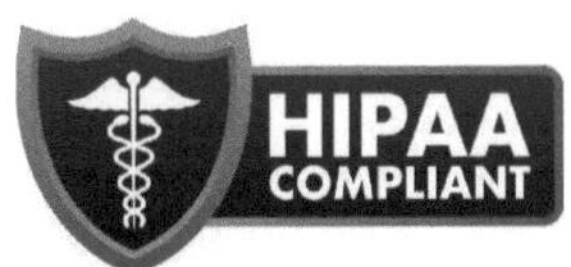

The Health Insurance Portability and Accountability Act

قاعدة حفظ الخصوصيات التابعة لقانون إخضاع التأمين الصحي لقابلية النقل والمحاسبية

The Health Insurance Portability and Accountability Act of 1996 (HIPAA)

HIPAA is the acronym for the Health Insurance Portability and Accountability Act of 1996. The Centers for Medicare & Medicaid Services (CMS) are responsible for implementing various unrelated provisions of HIPAA, therefore HIPAA may mean different things to different people. Here's a directory of CMS's business activities with regards to HIPAA.

HIPAA Health Insurance Reform

Title I of the Health Insurance Portability and Accountability Act of 1996 (HIPAA) protects health insurance coverage for workers and their families when they change or lose their jobs.

HIPAA Administrative Simplification

The Administrative Simplification provisions of the Health Insurance Portability and Accountability Act of 1996 (HIPAA, Title II) require the Department of Health and Human Services to establish national standards for electronic health care transactions and national identifiers for providers, health plans, and employers. It also addresses the security and privacy of health data. Adopting these standards will improve the efficiency and effectiveness of the nation's health care system by encouraging the widespread use of electronic data interchange in health care.

Overview

The Health Insurance Portability and Accountability Act of 1996, known as HIPAA, includes important new - but limited - protections for millions of working Americans and their families. HIPAA may:

1. Increase your ability to get health coverage for yourself and your dependents if you start a new job;
2. Lower your chance of losing existing health care coverage, whether you have that coverage through a job, or through individual health insurance;
3. Help you maintain continuous health coverage for yourself and your dependents when you change jobs; and
4. Help you buy health insurance coverage on your own if you lose coverage under an employer's group health plan and have no other health coverage available.

Among its specific protections, HIPAA:
1. Limits the use of pre-existing condition exclusions;
2. Prohibits group health plans from discriminating by denying you coverage or charging you extra for coverage based on your or your family member's past or present poor health;
3. Guarantees certain small employers, and certain individuals who lose job-related coverage, the right to purchase health insurance and;
4. Guarantees, in most cases, that employers or individuals who purchase health insurance can renew the coverage
Regardless of any health conditions on the individuals covered under the insurance policy.

In short, HIPAA may lower your chance of losing existing coverage, ease your ability to switch health plans and/or help you buy coverage on your own if you lose your employer's plan and have no other coverage available.

HIPAA Compliance – What Medical Interpreters Need to Know
When a health care provider covered by the Health Insurance Portability and Accountability Act (HIPAA) uses an interpreter to communicate with an individual, that individual's authorization is not required for the disclosure of protected health information to the interpreter, as long as certain conditions are met.

Since medical interpreters are the communication middle ground between patients and doctors, they certainly interact with this type of information in the course of their job and are therefore required to be HIPAA compliant.

HIPAA compliance is crucial for all healthcare providers. It ensures the facility follows all of the rules regarding patient privacy, which is essential.

In the world of patient care, medical interpreters are a critical part of the equation. About 35 million U.S. citizens who are over the age of 18 don't speak English at home. That's more than 15 percent of the population. While some of those 35 million adults do speak English very well, many don't. That's why medical interpreters are so vital.

As a medical interpreter, you also have a responsibility to maintain patient privacy. If you are wondering how the HIPAA rules impact you, here's what you need to know.

What Is HIPAA?
HIPAA is an acronym that stands for "Health Insurance Portability and Accountability Act." It's a federal law – overseen by the U.S. Department of Health and Human Services (HHS) Office for Civil Rights – that outlines the proper treatment of patient information, which is labeled as Protected Health Information (**PHI**).

In the simplest sense, HIPAA requires medical professionals – including medical interpreters – to safeguard patient data. This includes in communications – both verbal and in writing – as those can contain patient details that need to be protected.

What Qualifies as PHI?

A variety of patient details fall in the PHI category. Personally identifiable information (PII) – including names, addresses, phone numbers, dates of birth, demographic classifications, Social Security Numbers, and more – are all part of the PHI group.

Additionally, many health details qualify as PHI. This includes:
- Past, present, or future medical concerns or diagnoses, including physical and mental health conditions
- Appointment schedules
- Provider names
- Treatment types
- Test results, and more

Essentially, most patient details are protected, even if they seem small or inconsequential.

How HIPAA Violations Impact Medical Interpreters

Above all, HIPAA protects patient privacy. As a medical interpreter, you have to treat all patient information correctly. Otherwise, you are not HIPAA compliant. The penalties for a HIPAA violation can be incredibly severe. Violations can come with steep fines as well as criminal charges. While willful violations come with the steepest penalties – including up to a $50,000 to $100,000 per violation fine and up to five years in prison – even unknowing or 'reasonable cause' violations have penalties. You could still see fines up to $50,000 per violation, even if the incident was accidental and not willful.

How to Remain HIPAA Compliant as a Medical Interpreter

Here's a look at what medical interpreters need to do to remain HIPAA compliant.

- Do not Discuss Patient Details with Anyone Who Isn't Directly Involved with the Patient

As a medical interpreter, you need to ensure that you do not reveal any patient details to anyone who isn't directly involved with the patient. This means limiting communication to only pre-approved individuals on the medical team and pre-authorized family members or friends. If you need to share information with an approved individual, you must do so only if others can't overhear the discussion. Usually, this means entering a private space and closing the door.

- Exercise Caution When Using Unprotected Emails, Messaging Systems, or Phone or Video Call Systems

Unprotected email and messaging systems, as well as phone or video call technologies, aren't inherently secure. As a result, you need to make sure you do not reveal certain patient details when using those communication tools, ensuring the patient's privacy if the message or call is intercepted by an unauthorized party.

- Avoid using the patient's full name or revealing PII that could lead to the patient's identity.

Limit the sharing of medical details that could make the patient known to others as well.

- Properly Dispose of or Store Paper That Contains PHI

If you end up with documents or take notes that contain any PHI, make sure they are stored or disposed of in accordance with HIPAA policy. For example, this can mean using only approved storage mechanisms – both physical and digital – or a HIPAA-compliant shredder, depending on whether the paperwork needs to be maintained.

Like many regulations, patient privacy laws can change, as well as vary by location. States may enact more requirements, or new federal policies may make process changes necessary. For example, the Health Information Technology for Economic Clinical Health (HITECH) Act serves as a supplement to HIPAA. It outlines additional requirements regarding the use of technology by healthcare providers and, since online communication platforms are increasingly common, can impact medical interpreters.

Code of Ethics for Interpreters in Healthcare

- The interpreter treats as confidential, within the treating team; all information learned in the performance of their professional duties, while observing relevant requirements regarding disclosure.
- The interpreter strives to render the message accurately, conveying the content and spirit of the original message, taking into consideration its cultural context.
- The interpreter strives to maintain impartiality and refrains from counseling, advising or projecting personal biases or beliefs.
- The interpreter maintains the boundaries of the professional role, refraining from personal involvement.
- The interpreter continuously strives to develop awareness of his/her own and other (including biomedical) cultures encountered in the performance of their professional duties. The interpreter treats all parties with respect.
- When the patient's health, well-being, or dignity is at risk, the interpreter may be justified in acting as an advocate. Advocacy is understood as an action taken on behalf of an individual that goes beyond facilitating communication, with the intention of supporting good health outcomes. Advocacy must only be undertaken after careful and thoughtful analysis of the situation and if other less intrusive actions have not resolved the problem.
- The interpreter strives to continually further his/her knowledge and skills. The interpreter must, at all times, act in a professional and ethical manner.

Roles of an interpreter

There are 4 roles as below:

1. **CONDUIT** :

In this role, the interpreter acts as a means for what is said by one party to reach the other. This is the basic or default role of the interpreter. The interpreter speaks what has been said in the other language, BECOMING THE VOICE OF THE PATIENT AND THE PROVIDER.

2. **CLARIFIER** :

There are times when a term or phrase is not heard or understood. Usually evidenced by a "blank stare" or a delay in the response to a question. In this role, the interpreter checks for understanding and seeks to remove any doubts about what was said. The interpreter assumes this role when they believe it is necessary to facilitate understanding.

3. **CULTURAL BROKER or CULTURAL INTERFACE**:

Taking on this role implies having knowledge on the particular cultural beliefs of the individuals you are interpreting for. That knowledge of different cultures allows the interpreter to detect cultural misunderstandings and assume the role of cultural interface, providing the necessary cultural framework to clear up any misunderstanding.

4. **ADVOCATE** :

In this role, the interpreter goes beyond being the patient's voice. Here the interpreter ACTS on certain issues that they feel are necessary for the patient to get the appropriate care he needs. THE INTERPRETER IS CONCERNED ABOUT THE QUALITY OF CARE that the LEP patient is to receive. It is the most "active" role an interpreter can assume and usually the least frequent one.

There is a lot of controversy over how much an interpreter should become involved in the patient's healthcare needs. The general consensus is that this role should be assumed by the interpreter TO AVOID HARM TO THE PATIENT OR ANOTHER PARTY.

With each role the interpreter's participation increases (incremental intervention). The interpreter's participation is minimal in the role of conduit and maximal in the role of advocate. The interpreter should always assume the least invasive role that will permit effective communication.

English – Arabic Glossary of some Healthcare professionals

	Healthcare Proffesional	مزاولي المهن الصحية
1	Doctor / physician	دكتور / طبيب
2	General practioner (GP)	طبيب عام
3	Specialist	إختصاصي
4	Consultant	استشاري
5	Surgeon	جراح
6	Technician	فني – تقني
7	Nurse	ممرض
	Registered Nurse	ممرض مسجل
8	Assistant Nurse	مساعد ممرض
9	Nurse Practitioner	ممرض ممارس
10	Aesthetician	فني تجميل
11	Allergist/immunologist	أختصاصي الحساسية / المناعة
12	Anesthesiologist	طبيب التخدير
13	Audiologist	أخصائي السمع
14	Bariatric and obesity surgeon	جراح السمنة (إنقاص الوزن)
15	Cardiologist	طبيب القلب
16	Dermatologist	طبيب الجلدية
17	Dentist	طبيب أسنان
18	Endocrinologist	طبيب الغدد الصماء
19	Family physician	طبيب الأسرة
20	Gastroenterologist	طبيب الجهاز الهضمي
21	Geneticist	اختصاصي علوم الوراثة
22	Geriatrist	طبيب الشيخوخة (كبار العمر)
23	Health Educator	مثقف صحي
24	Hematologist	طبيب أمراض الدم
25	Hospice and palliative medicine specialist	إختصاصي رعاية المسنين والطب التلطيفي
26	Infectious disease physician	طبيب الأمراض المعدية
27	Internal Medicine	الطب الباطني

28	Medical Transcriptionist	ناسخ طبي
29	Nephrologist	طبيب أمراض الكلى
30	Neurologist	طبيب أعصاب
31	Obstetrician/gynecologist (OBGYNs)	طبيب التوليد / أمراض النساء
32	Occupational therapist	إختصاصي العلاج الوظيفي
33	Occupational health physician	طبيب الصحة المهنية
34	Oncologist	طبيب الأورام
35	Ophthalmologist	إختصاصي بصريات
36	Optometrist	طبيب العيون
37	Orthopedist	طبيب عظام
38	Otolaryngologist	طبيب أنف وأذن وحنجرة
39	Osteopath	طبيب العظام
40	Paramedic	إختصاصي طب طوارئ
41	Pathologist	إختصاصي علم الأمراض
42	Pediatrician	طبيب الأطفال
43	Physiotherapist	معالج طبيعي
44	Phlebotomist	فني سحب دم
45	Plastic surgeon	جراح تجميل
46	Podiatrist	معالج القدم
47	Psychiatrist	طبيب نفسي
48	Pulmonologist	طبيب الرئة
49	Radiologist	إختصاصي أشعة
50	Rheumatologist	طبيب روماتيزم
51	Sleep medicine specialist	إختصاصي طب اضطرابات النوم
52	Sonographer	إختصاصي التصوير بالأمواج فوق الصوتية
53	Surgeon	دكتور جراح
54	Urologist	طبيب مسالك بولية

Section 2

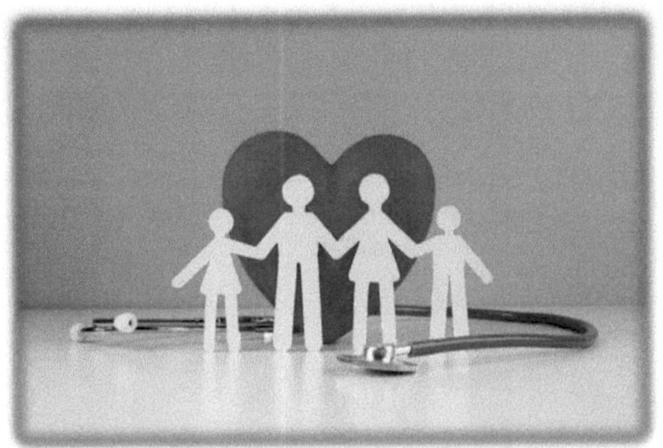

Chapter One- Anatomy & Physiology

Overview

This chapter introduces the reader to common medical terminology of Anatomy and Physiology that will include bilingual terminology for the following;

1. Anatomy
2. Common Symptoms
3. Common Diseases and disorders
4. Investigations
5. Common Vaccines

We hope you enjoy reading this Chapter, and more chapters awaiting you

Human Muscle Anatomy

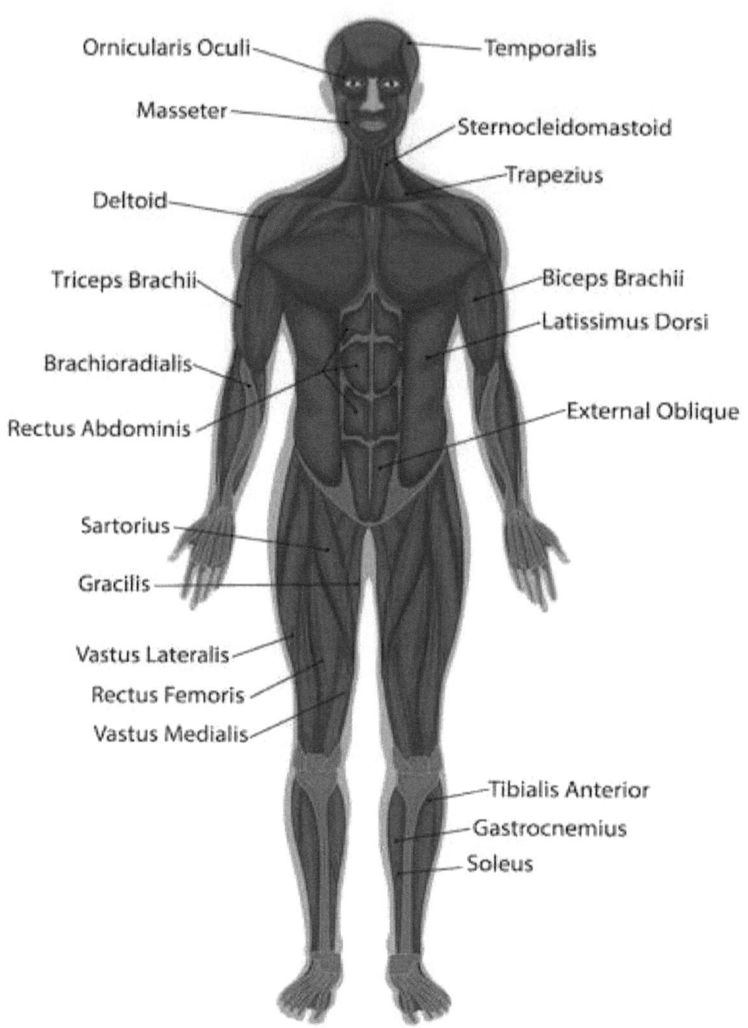

Human anatomy

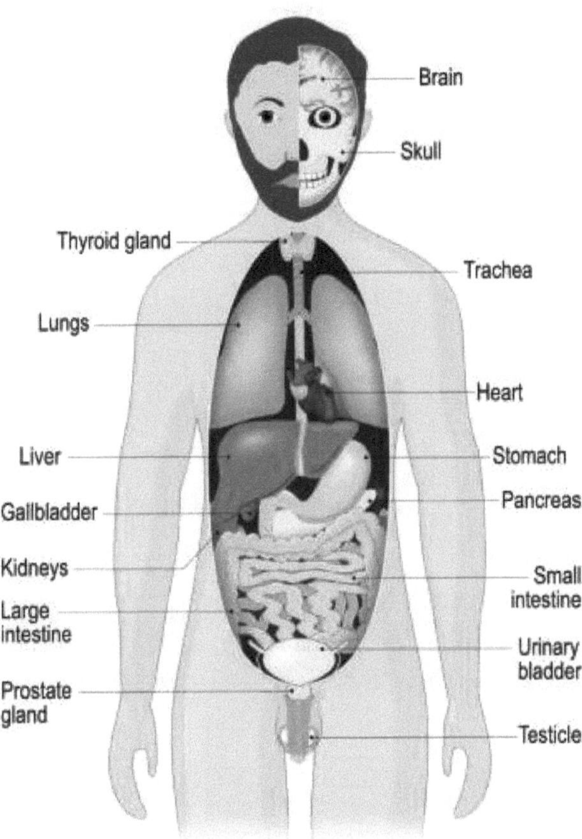

HUMAN SKELETON

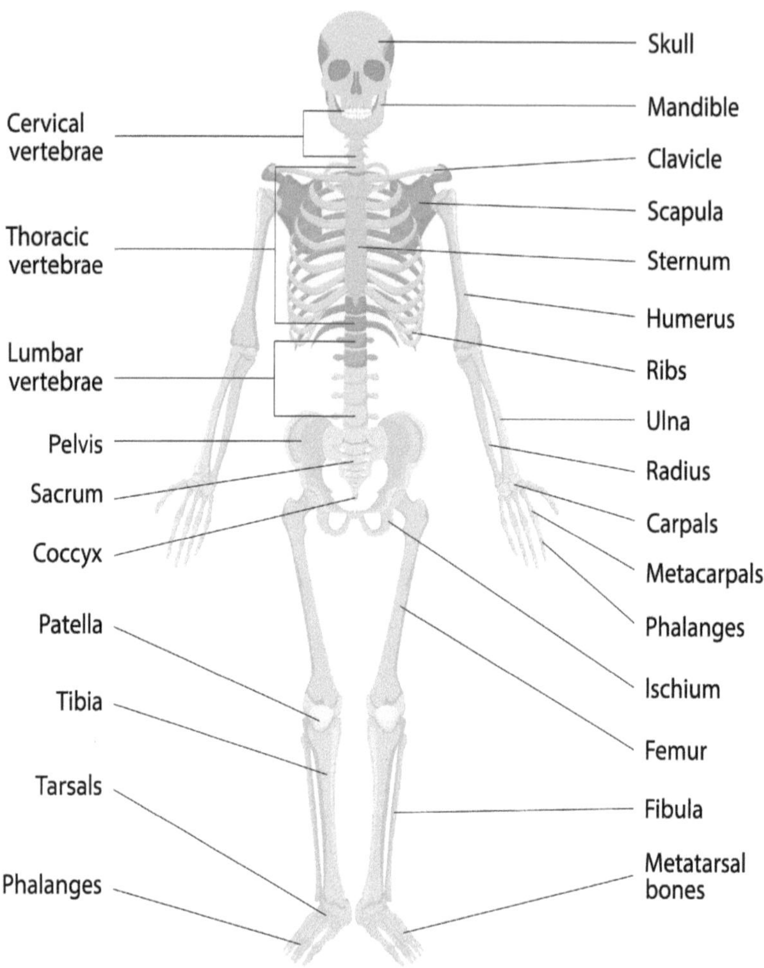

There are 11 major organ systems in the human body:	
1	Skeletal System	الجهاز الهيكلي العظمي
2	Muscular System	الجهاز العضلي
3	Cardiovascular System	الجهاز القلبي الوعائي
4	Nervous system	الجهاز العصبي
5	Lymphatic System	الجهاز اللمفاوي
6	Respiratory System	الجهاز التنفسي
7	Digestive System	الجهاز الهضمي
8	Urinary System	الجهاز البولي
9	Reproductive system	الجهاز التناسلي
10	The integumentary system	الجهاز اللحافي (الغلافي)
11	The endocrine system	نظام الغدد الصماء
12	The immune system	الجهاز المناعي

An organ system is a group of organs that work together in the body to perform a complex function, such as pumping blood or processing and utilizing nutrients. There are 11 major organ systems in the human body:

	The organ system	Organs	Description
1	**The circulatory system**	• Heart • Blood vessels (arteries and veins) The blood itself	The circulatory system transports oxygen and nutrients to all corners of the body. It also carries away carbon dioxide and other waste products.
	الجهاز الدوري **(الدورة الدموية)**	• قلب • الأوعية الدموية (الشرايين والأوردة)	يقوم الجهاز الدوري بنقل الأكسجين والمواد المغذية إلى جميع أنحاء الجسم. كما أنها تنقل ثاني أكسيد الكربون ومنتجات المخلفات الأخرى.
2	**The lymphatic system**	• **Lymph vessels** • **Lymph nodes** • **Lymph ducts** • **Various glands**	**The lymphatic system is the drainage system of the body. It plays an important role in your immunity, blood pressure regulation, digestion, and other**

functions.

الجهاز اللمفاوي

- الأوعية الليمفاوية
- الغدد الليمفاوية
- القنوات الليمفاوية
- الغدد المختلفة

الجهاز اللمفاوي هو نظام تصريف الجسم. يلعب دورًا مهمًا في المناعة وتنظيم ضغط الدم والهضم والوظائف الأخرى.

3 **The respiratory system**

- Lungs
- Trachea (windpipe)
- Airways of the respiratory tree

The respiratory system is responsible for breathing, which is the controlled movement of air in and out of the body (ventilation). It also moves oxygen and carbon dioxide into and out of the bloodstream (respiration).

الجهاز التنفسي

- الرئتين
- القصبة الهوائية
- تفريعات المجاري التنفسية

الجهاز التنفسي مسؤول عن التنفس، وهو التحكم في حركة الهواء داخل وخارج الجسم (التهوية). كما أنه ينقل الأكسجين وثاني أكسيد الكربون داخل وخارج مجرى الدم (التنفس).

4	**The integumentary system**	The integumentary system is the skin and all the structures in it, including the: • Sweat glands • Hair follicles • Nails • Nerves	The integumentary system is unique because it is the largest and only single-organ system in the body. It protects the body from the external environment and helps regulate body temperature.
	الجهاز اللحافي (الغلافي)	نظام غلافي هو الجلد وجميع مكوناته، بما في ذلك: • الغدد العرقية • بصيلات الشعر • الأظافر • الأعصاب	نظام غلافي فريد من نوعه لأنه أكبر نظام وحيد العضو في الجسم. يحمي الجسم من البيئة الخارجية ويساعد في تنظيم درجة حرارة الجسم .
5	**The endocrine system**	This organ system includes all the glands that secrete hormones into the bloodstream, including:5 • Adrenal • Gonads (ovaries and testicles) • Hypothalamus • Pancreas • Pineal • Pituitary • Thymus • Thyroid • Parathyroid	The endocrine system mostly regulates metabolism and uses the products of digestion. Along with the nervous system and immune system, it's generally considered one of the most complicated systems in the body.
	نظام الغدد الصماء	يشمل هذا الجهاز جميع الغدد التي تفرز الهرمونات في مجرى الدم ومنها: • الغدة الكظرية • الغدد التناسلية (المبايض والخصيتين) • تحت المهاد • البنكرياس • الصنوبرية • الغدة النخامية • الغدة الزعترية • الغدة الدرقية • جار درقية	في الغالب ينظم جهاز الغدد الصماء عملية التمثيل الغذائي ويستخدم منتجات الهضم. إلى جانب الجهاز العصبي والجهاز المناعي ، يعتبر بشكل عام أحد أكثر الأجهزة تعقيدًا في الجسم.

<table>
<tr><td>

6

The gastrointestinal (digestive) system

</td><td>

- Mouth
- Esophagus
- Stomach
- Small intestine
- Large intestine
- Rectum
- Anus
- The pancreas
- gallbladder
- liver.

</td><td>

The gastrointestinal (GI) system is sometimes referred to as the gut or the digestive system. It is responsible for breaking down foods into nutrients, which the body needs for energy, growth, and cell repair. This system includes all the organs that carry food from where it enters the body to where it exits, including the

</td></tr>
</table>

الجهاز الهضمي	يشمل هذا النظام جميع الأعضاء التي تحمل الطعام من حيث يدخل الجسم إلى حيث يخرج منها: • الفم • المريء • المعدة • الأمعاء الدقيقة • الأمعاء الغليظة • المستقيم • فتحة الشرج • البنكرياس • المرارة • الكبد.	يشار أحيانًا إلى الجهاز الهضمي (GI) باسم القناة الهضمية أو الجهاز الهضمي. وهو مسؤول عن تفتيت الأطعمة إلى عناصر غذائية يحتاجها الجسم للطاقة والنمو وإصلاح الخلايا. يشمل هذا النظام جميع الأعضاء التي تحمل الطعام من مكان دخوله إلى الجسم حتى خروجه، بما في ذلك الجهاز الهضمي

7	The urinary (excretory) system	<ul><li>Kidneys</li><li>Ureters</li><li>Bladder</li><li>Urethra</li></ul>	These organs work together to filter blood and remove toxins and waste from body tissues. The removal of excess fluid through this organ system also helps regulate blood pressure.

المسالك البولية (جهاز الإخراج)	• الكلى • الحالب • المثانة البولية • الإحليل	تعمل هذه الأعضاء معًا لتصفية الدم وإزالة السموم والفضلات من أنسجة الجسم. يساعد التخلص من السوائل الزائدة من خلال هذا الجهاز العضوي أيضًا على تنظيم ضغط الدم.

8	The musculoskeletal system	<ul><li>Skeleton</li><li>All the muscles, tendons, and ligaments attached to the skeleton</li></ul>The three types of muscles in the body are:<ul><li>Skeletal (voluntary)</li><li>Smooth (visceral or involuntary), which are inside walls of organs like the intestines</li><li>Cardiac (heart muscle)</li></ul>	The musculoskeletal system provides the framework and the engine for our movement, posture, and physical abilities.

الجهاز العضلي الهيكلي	• الهيكل العظمي • جميع العضلات والأوتار والأربطة المتصلة بالهيكل العظمي • أنواع العضلات الثلاثة في الجسم هي: • العضلات الهيكلية (الإرادية) • ملساء (حشوي أو اللاإرادية)، وهو موجود داخل جدران الأعضاء مثل الأمعاء • العضلات القلبية (عضلة القلب)	يوفر الجهاز العضلي الهيكلي الإطار والمحرك لحركتنا ووقفتنا وقدراتنا البدنية.

| 9 | **The nervous system** | - Brain
- Spinal cord
- All the nerves connected to both of these organs | The nervous system is a network that makes it possible for different parts of the body to communicate with one another. Think of it as your body's command station. All body processes, reactions, thoughts, and movements stem from this organ system. |

الجهاز العصبي

- المخ
- الحبل الشوكي
- جميع الأعصاب المتصلة بهذين العضوين

الجهاز العصبي عبارة عن شبكة تتيح لأجزاء مختلفة من الجسم التواصل مع بعضها البعض. فكر في الأمر كمركز قيادة لجسدك. جميع عمليات الجسم وردود الفعل والأفكار والحركات تنبع من هذا الجهاز العضوي.

| 10 | **The reproductive system** | The male reproductive system includes the:

- Penis
- Testicles

The female reproductive system includes the:15

- Vagina
- Uterus
- Ovaries | This is the only organ system that is not complete in any one body and requires another person (or medical intervention) to complete its mission, which is to produce offspring. |

الجهاز التناسلي

يشمل الجهاز التناسلي الذكري:

- القضيب
- الخصيتين

يشمل الجهاز التناسلي الأنثوي:

- المهبل
- رَحِم
- المبايض

هذا هو الجهاز الوحيد الذي لا يكتمل في أي جسم ويتطلب شخصًا آخر (أو تدخلًا طبيًا) لإكمال مهمته، وهي التناسل.

| 11 | The immune system | • Lymph nodes
• Bone marrow
• Thymus
• Spleen
• Adenoids
• Tonsils
• Skin | The immune system helps the body fight against infection and other diseases. It is listed last because, while it's important for survival, all of its organs are borrowed from other organ systems. |

| 12 | الجهاز المناعي | • الغدد الليمفاوية
• نخاع العظم
• الغدة الزعترية
• طحال
• اللحمية
• اللوزتين
• الجلد | يساعد جهاز المناعة الجسم على مقاومة العدوى والأمراض الأخرى. تم إدراجه أخيرًا لأنه على الرغم من أهميته للبقاء على قيد الحياة ، يتم استعارة جميع أعضائه من أنظمة أعضاء أخرى. |

Common symptoms

Term	المصطلح
Common Symptoms	
Skeletal system	الجهاز الهيكلي
bone pain – Joint pain – Muscle pain	آلام العظام, آلام المفصل, آلام العضلات
fractures from low impact, low energy activities	الكسور من الأنشطة ذات التأثير المنخفض وانخفاض الطاقة, آلام الوتر والأربطة
tendon and ligament pain	
sprains - swelling	الالتواء ـ الانتفاخات (التورمات)
infections - inflammation	العدوى – الالتهابات
joint pain	الم المفاصل
back pain	ألم في الظهر
weakness	ضعف
Aching and stiffness.	وجع وتيبس.
Burning sensations in the muscles.	حرقان في العضلات.
Fatigue.	تعب.
Muscle spasm	تشنجات العضلات.
Pain that worsens with movement.	ألم يزداد سوءًا مع الحركة.
Sleep disturbances.	اضطرابات النوم.
Muscular system	الجهاز العضلي
Muscle weakness that can lead to cramps, aches and pains.	ضعف العضلات الذي يمكن أن يؤدي إلى ارتعاش وتشنجات وآلام.
Muscle wasting	هزال العضلات.
Movement issues.	مشاكل في الحركة.
Balance problems.	مشاكل التوازن.
Numbness, tingling or painful sensations.	تنميل أو وخز أو إحساس مؤلم.
Droopy eyelids.	ترهل الجفون.
Double vision.	ازدواجية في الرؤية
Trouble swallowing.	صعوبة في البلع.

Abnormal gait	مشية غير طبيعية

Cardiovascular system	الجهاز القلبي الوعائي
pain, weakness or numb legs and/or arms.	ألم أو ضعف أو خدر في الساقين و / أو الذراعين.
breathlessness.	ضيق التنفس.
very fast or slow heartbeat, or palpitations.	ضربات قلب سريعة جدًا أو بطيئة ، أو خفقان القلب.
feeling dizzy, lightheaded or faint.	الشعور بالدوار أو خفة في الرأس أو الإغماء.
fatigue.	تعب.
swollen limbs.	تورم الأطراف.
Chest pain (angina).	ألم في الصدر (الذبحة الصدرية).
Chest pressure, heaviness or discomfort, sometimes described as a "belt around the chest" or a "weight on the chest."	ضغط على الصدر أو ثقله أو عدم الارتياح ، ويوصف أحيانًا بأنه "حزام حول الصدر" أو "ثقل على الصدر".
Shortness of breath (dyspnea).	ضيق التنفس.
Dizziness or fainting.	دوار أو إغماء.
Fatigue or exhaustion.	التعب أو الإرهاق.
Pain or cramps in your legs when you walk.	ألم أو تقلصات في ساقيك عند المشي.
Leg sores that aren't healing.	تقرحات الساق التي لا تلتئم.
Cool or red skin on your legs.	برودة أو احمرار على الساق
Swelling in your legs. Ankle swelling	تورم في الساق. تورم في الكاحل
Numbness in your face or a limb. This may be on only one side of your body.	خدر في وجهك أو أحد أطرافك. قد يكون هذا في جانب واحد فقط من جسمك.
Difficulty with talking, seeing or walking.	صعوبة في الكلام أو الرؤية أو المشي.

Nervous system	الجهاز العصبي
Persistent or sudden onset of a headache	صداع مستمر أو مفاجئ
A headache that changes or is different	صداع متغير أو بحالات مختلفة
Loss of feeling or tingling	فقدان الإحساس أو الوخز
Weakness or loss of muscle strength / paralysis	ضعف أو فقدان قوة العضلات / الشلل
Loss of sight or double vision	فقدان البصر أو ازدواج في الرؤية

Memory loss	فقدان الذاكرة
Impaired mental ability	ضعف القدرة العقلية
Lack of coordination	ضعف التنسيق
Muscle rigidity	تصلب العضلات
Tremors and seizures	الرعشات والنوبات
Back pain which radiates to the feet, toes, or other parts of the body	آلام الظهر التي تنتشر في القدمين أو أصابع القدم أو أجزاء أخرى من الجسم
Muscle wasting and slurred speech	ضعف العضلات وتداخل الكلام
New language impairment (expression or comprehension)	اعاقة لغوية حديثة (التعبير أو الفهم)
Vision problems or headaches.	مشاكل في الرؤية أو صداع.
Slurred speech.	اللعثمة في الكلام (كلام غير مفهوم)
Numbness, tingling, or loss of sensation in your arms or legs.	خدر أو وخز أو فقدان الإحساس في ذراعيك أو ساقيك.
Tremors or tics (random muscle movements).	الرعشات أو التشنجات اللاإرادية (حركات العضلات العشوائية).
Changes in behavior or memory.	التغييرات في السلوك أو الذاكرة.
Problems with coordination or moving your muscles.	مشاكل في التنسيق أو تحريك عضلاتك.
Lymphatic system	الجهاز اللمفاوي
swelling of lymph nodes in your neck, armpits or groin	تورم في الغدد الليمفاوية في رقبتك أو الإبط أو الفخذ
Persistent fatigue	التعب المستمر
Fever	حمى
Night sweats	تعرق ليلي
Shortness of breath	ضيق في التنفس
Unexplained weight loss	فقدان الوزن غير المبرر
Itchy skin	حكة في الجلد
Swelling of part or all of the arm or leg, including fingers or toes	تورم في جزء أو كل الذراع أو الساق ، بما في ذلك أصابع اليدين أو القدمين

A feeling of heaviness or tightness	الشعور بالثقل أو الضيق
Restricted range of motion	محدودية في نطاق الحركة
Recurring infections	عدوى متكررة
Hardening and thickening of the skin (fibrosis)	تصلب الجلد وتثخنه (تليف)

Respiratory System	الجهاز التنفسي
Sneezing	العطس
a stuffy or runny nose	انسداد أو سيلان الأنف
Wheezing	صفير
Chest tightness	ضيق في الصدر
headaches	الصداع
muscle aches	آلام العضلات
breathlessness, tight chest or wheezing	ضيق في التنفس أو ضيق في الصدر أو أزيز
a high temperature	ارتفاع حرارة الجسم
feeling generally unwell	الشعور بتوعك بشكل عام
Fever.	حمى.
Hoarse voice.	صوت أجش.
Fatigue and lack of energy.	التعب وقلة الطاقة.
Red eyes.	احمرار العيون
Runny nose.	سيلان الأنف.
Sore throat.	إلتهاب الحلق.
Swollen lymph nodes (swelling on the sides of your neck).	تورم الغدد الليمفاوية (تورم على جانبي رقبتك).

Digestive System	الجهاز الهضمي
GERD (Gastroesophageal Reflux Disease)	GERD (مرض الارتجاع المعدي المريئي) الارتجاع المعدي المريئي
Acid Reflux	ارتجاع الحمض المريئي
Burning sensation	إحساس بالحرقان
Bloating	انتفاخ

Constipation	امساك
Diarrhea	إسهال
Abdominal pain	وجع في البطن
Nausea	غثيان، لوعة
Peptic Ulcer Disease	مرض القرحة الهضمية
Loss of appetite	فقدان الشهية
Miscellaneous	متنوع
Back pain	ألم في الظهر
Ear discharge	افرازات الأذن
Flank pain	الم الخاصرة
Flu	رشح، زكام
Vertigo	دوار
Back pain	الم الظهر
Malaise/fatigue	إعياء تعب
Sciatica pain	الم العصب الوركي (عرق النسا)
Diabetic neuropathy	اعتلال اعصاب سكري
Syncope	اغماء
Confusion	التباس، ارتباك، التشوش
Vomiting	تقيؤ
Renal insufficiency	قصور كلوي
Fluid retention	احتباس سوائل
Shortness of breath	قصر النفس
Irregular heartbeat	عدم انتظام نبضات القلب
Chronic bronchitis	التهاب رئوي مزمن
Wheezing	صفير
Mucus	مخاط
Chest Tightness	ضيق بالصدر
Inflammation	التهاب

Obesity	السمنة
Asthma	ربو
Fatty liver disease	امراض الكبد الدهني
High cholesterol	ارتفاع الكوليسترول
Sleep apnea	انقطاع النفس اثناء النوم
Arthritis	التهاب المفاصل
Infertility	العقم
Hormonal imbalances	اختلال التوازن الهرموني
Complications	مضاعفات
Vitamin deficiencies	نقص فيتامينات
Thirst	عطش
Hunger	جوع
Irritability	التهيج
Blurred vision	تشوش الرؤية
Breath odor	رائحة النفس
Tingling	تنميل
Numbness	خدران
Fever	حمى
Eczema	جلدي مرض الاكزيما
Constipation	إمساك
Depression	اكتئاب
Tobacco abuse	تعاطي التبغ
Sore throat	إلتهاب الحلق
Shingles	هربس نطاقي (حزام ناري)
Rashes	الطفح الجلدي
Heartburn	حرقة في المعدة
Insomnia	أرق
Anxiety	قلق

Sinusitis	التهاب الجيوب الأنفية
Migraine	صداع نصفي (الشقيقة)
Developmental delays	تأخر النمو
Erectile dysfunction	الضعف الجنسي لدى الرجال
Degeneration	تنكس (خشونة)
Abuse	افراط -إساءة استخدام
Trauma	صدمة / إصابة
Functional decline	تدهور وظيفي
hypertension	ارتفاع ضغط الدم
Hearing loss	فقدان السمع
Suicidal thoughts	أفكار انتحارية
Aches and pains	اوجاع والآم
Balance disorder	اضطراب التوازن
Fall risk	خطر السقوط
Dementia	الخَرَف
Headache	صداع

Diseases/Health Conditions

Disease/health conditions	
Term	المصطلح
1	Cognitive impairment	الضعف الادراكي (الاختلال المعرفي)
2	Chronic obstructive pulmonary disease (COPD)	مرض الانسداد الرئوي المزمن
3	Endocrine disorders	امراض الغدد الصم
4	Diabetes	السكري
5	Prediabetes	مرحلة ماقبل السكري
6	Gestational diabetes	سكر الحمل
7	Hypoglycemia	هبوط سكر الدم
8	Hyperglycemia	ارتفاع سكر الدم
9	Hemoglobin A1C (hba1c)	السكر التراكمي (الهيموجلبين A1C)
10	Insulin shock	غيبوبة بسبب فقد الانسولين
11	Gangrene	الغرغرينة
12	Polycystic ovary syndrome (PCOS)	متلازمة المبيض متعدد الكيسات
13	Cushing syndrome	متلازمة كوشينغ
14	Hyperthyroidism	فرط نشاط الغدة الدرقية
15	Hypothyroidism	قصور الغدة درقية
16	Goiter	تضخم غدة درقية (مرض غويتر)
17	Osteoarthritis	التهاب المفاصل الروماتيزمي
18	Stroke	سكته دماغي
19	Gallbladder	المرارة
20	Fatty liver disease	امراض الكبد الدهني
21	High cholesterol	ارتفاع الكوليسترول
22	DVT Deep Vein Thrombosis	تجلط الأوردة العميقة
23	Clot/Thrombus	جلطة دموية
24	Atherosclerosis	تصلب الشرايين

25	Transient ischemic attack (TIA)	نوبة نقص تروية عابرة
26	Peripheral Artery Disease (PAD)	مرض الشريان المحيطي
27	Peripheral Vascular Disease or PVD	مرض الوعاء المحيطي
28	Varicose Veins	الدوالي
29	Spider veins	عروق العنكبوت
30	Renal failure	فشل كلوي
31	Hyperkalaemia	ارتفاع البوتاسيوم في الدم
32	Inflammation	التهاب
33	Ketoacidosis DKA	الحماض الكيتوني السكري
34	Thyroid Disorders	امراض الغدة الدرقية
35	Increased metabolic rate	ازدياد معدل الاستقلاب (التمثيل الغذائي/الأيض)
	Grave's disease	مرض غرايفز
	Hashimoto disease	داءُ هاشيموتو
	Discharge	الافرازات
	Endocarditis	التهاب بطانة القلب
	Pneumonia	التهاب الرئة
	Urinary tract infection	التهاب المسالك البولية
	Cellulitis	التهاب النسيج الخلوي
	Sexually transmitted infections	الامراض المنتقلة جنسيا
	Tuberculosis (TB)	الدرن/السل

Investigations

Investigations	
Diagnostic Services	
Laboratory	
Blood Urea Nitrogen	نيتروجين يوريا الدم
Creatinine	الكرياتينين
Electrolytes, such as potassium, phosphate, and sodium help carry electrical signals between cells.	تساعد الشوارد الكهارل (الأملاح)، مثل البوتاسيوم والفوسفات والصوديوم، في نقل الإشارات الكهربائية بين الخلايا.
Comprehensive Metabolic Panel	تحاليل الاستقلاب الشاملة
Lipid Panel	مجموعة تحاليل الدهون)الكوليسترول(
Total Cholesterol (TC)	الكوليسترول الكلي
High-density lipoprotein (HDL)	الدهون مرتفعة الكثافة (الكوليسترول النافع)
low-density lipoprotein (LDL)	الدهون منخفضة الكثافة (الكوليسترول الضار)
Triglycerides (TG)	الدهون الثلاثية
Liver function tests	اختبار وظائف الكبد
Kidney function tests	اختبار وظائف الكلية
Bilirubin	البيليروبين
Total protein	فحص البروتين الكامل
Albumin	الألبومين
C-reactive protein (CRP)	اختبار البروتين المتفاعل -C (فحص العامل الالتهابي)
Thyroid Stimulating Hormone	الهرمون المحفز للغدة الدرقية
Urinalysis	تحليل البول
Cultures	اختبار مزرعة
Radiology	
X-ray	اشعة سينية
Bone densitometry (DXA scan)	قياس كثافة العظام
Fluoroscopy	تنظير الفلور

Ultrasound	الموجات فوق الصوتية
Magnetic Resonance Imaging (MRI)	التصوير بالرنين المغناطيسي
Computed Tomography (CT)	التصوير المقطعي
Nuclear CT	التصوير النووي
Full body mole check	فحص الشامات الكامل الجسم
Mammogram	تصوير الثدي الشعاعي
Pap smear	اختبار عنق الرحم
EKG/ECG	مخطط كهربية القلب
electrocardiogram records the electrical signals in the heart	يسجل مخطط كهربية القلب الإشارات الكهربائية في القلب
Biopsy	خزعة

Common Vaccines

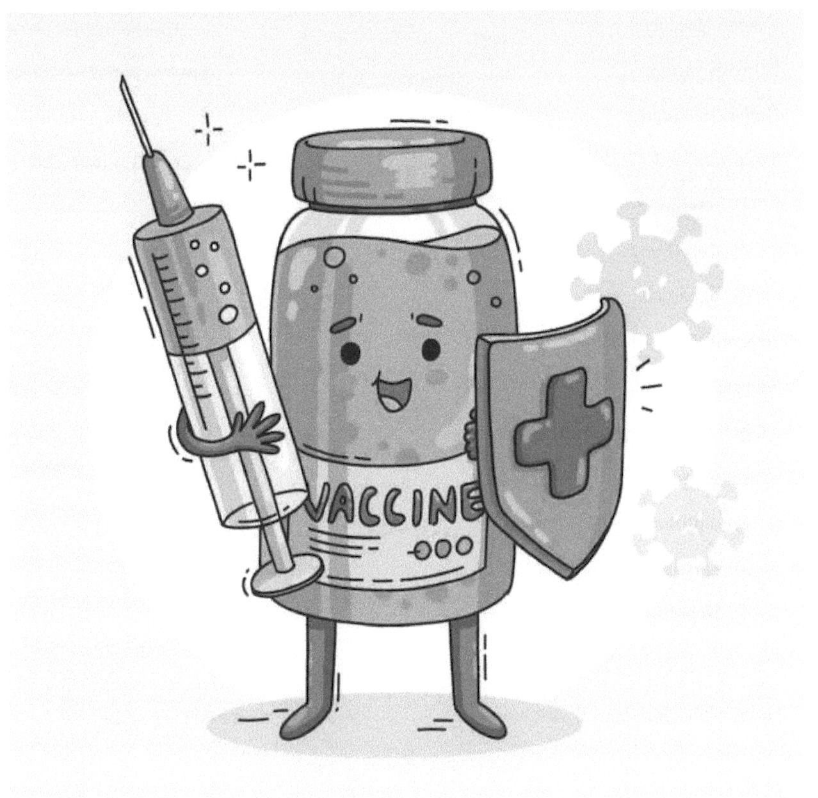

Common Vaccines

#	Vaccine	اسم التطعيم
	Tetanus Vaccine	تطعيم ضد الكزاز (التيتانوس)
	Pertussis vaccine	تطعيم ضد السعال الديكي (الشاهوق)
	Diphtheria vaccine	تطعيم ضد الخناق (الدفتيريا)
3	**Tdap** vaccine **3** 1) **tetanus,** 2) **diphtheria,** 3) **pertussis.**	**لقاح الثلاثي البكتيري 3** 1) تطعيم ضد الكزاز (التيتانوس) tetanus 2) تطعيم ضد الخناق (الدفتيريا) diphtheria 3) تطعيم ضد السعال الديكي (الشاهوق) pertusis
	Hepatitis B vaccine	تطعيم ضد التهاب الكبد الوبائي ب
4	**Tetravaccine** **Tdap** vaccine **3** + **Hepatitis B vaccine** 1) **tetanus,** 2) **diphtheria,** 3) **pertussis.** 4) **Hepatitis B vaccine**	**لقاح رباعي 4** **لقاح الثلاثي البكتيري 3 + التطعيم الخاص بالالتهاب الكبدي الوبائي ب** 1) تطعيم ضد الكزاز (التيتانوس) tetanus 2) تطعيم ضد الخناق (الدفتيريا) diphtheria 3) تطعيم ضد السعال الديكي (الشاهوق) pertusis 4) تطعيم ضد التهاب الكبد الوبائي ب Hepatitis B vaccine
	Heamophilus Influenza B vaccine	المستدمية النزلية من النوع ب (التطعيم ضد التهاب السحايا)
5	**pentavalent vaccine** **Tdap** vaccine **3** + **Hepatitis B vaccine** + **Heamophilus Influenza B vaccine** 1) **tetanus,** 2) **diphtheria,** 3) **pertussis.** 4) **Hepatitis B vaccine** 5) **Heamophilus Influenza B vaccine**	**لقاح خماسي 5** **لقاح الثلاثي البكتيري 3 + التطعيم الخاص بالالتهاب الكبدي الوبائي ب** 1) تطعيم ضد الكزاز (التيتانوس) tetanus 2) تطعيم ضد الخناق (الدفتيريا) diphtheria 3) تطعيم ضد السعال الديكي (الشاهوق) pertusis 4) تطعيم ضد التهاب الكبد الوبائي ب Hepatitis B vaccine 5) التطعيم ضد التهاب السحايا **Heamophilus Influenza B**

Polio vaccine	تطعيم ضد شلل الأطفال
hexavalent vaccine6	**لقاح سداسي 6**
Tdap vaccine 3 + Hepatitis B vaccine	**لقاح الثلاثي البكتيري 3 + التطعيم الخاص بالالتهاب الكبدي الوبائي ب**
+ Heamophilus Influenza B vaccine	+تطعيم ضد شلل الأطفال
+ Polio vaccine	

6

1) **tetanus,**

2) **diphtheria,**

3) **pertussis.**

4) **Hepatitis B vaccine**

5) **Heamophilus Influenza B vaccine**

6) **Polio vaccine**

1) تطعيم ضد الكزاز (التيتانوس) tetanus

2) تطعيم ضد الخناق (الدفتيريا) diphtheria

3) تطعيم ضد السعال الديكي (الشاهوق) pertusis

4) تطعيم ضد التهاب الكبد الوبائي ب   Hepatitis B vaccine

5) التطعيم ضد التهاب السحايا   **Heamophilus Influenza B**

6) تطعيم ضد شلل الأطفال

Chickenpox vaccine	تطعيم فاعل ضد جدري الماء (الحماق)
Chickenpox inactivated Vaccine	تطعيم خامل ضد جدري الماء (الحماق)
Pneumococcal vaccine	تطعيم ضد التهاب السحايا (التهاب الرئة)
Human Papilloma Virus (HPV) vaccine	تطعيم ضد سرطان عنق الرحم (الفيروس الحليمي البشري)
Influenza vaccine	تطعيم ضد الإنفلونزا
Polio SABIN vaccine	تطعيم سابين ضد شلل الأطفال
Measles Mumps and Rubella (MMR) vaccine	التطعيم ضد الحصبة، والنكاف، والحصبة الألمانية (المطعوم الثلاثي)
Rabies Immune Globulin vaccine	التطعيم الخامل ضد داء الكلب (السعار)
Inactivated Rabies Virus vaccine	التطعيم الفاعل ضد داء الكلب (السعار)
Hepatitis B Immunoglobulin vaccine	تطعيم خامل ضد التهاب الكبد الوبائي ب
Hepatitis A Vaccine	تطعيم ضد التهاب الكبد الوبائي أ
Inactivated hepatitis A vaccine	تطعيم خامل ضد التهاب الكبد الوبائي أ
Yellow Fever vaccine	تطعيم ضد الحمى الصفراء
Typhoid Fever vaccine	تطعيم ضد حمى التيفونيد أو الحمى التيفية (حمى التيفيد)
Rubella vaccine	تطعيم ضد الحصبة الألمانية، الحميراء (الروبيلا)

Measles Vaccine	تطعيم ضد الحصبة (بوحمرون)
Tick Borne Encephalitis vaccine	تطعيم ضد التهاب الدماغ المنقول بواسطة القراد
Japanese encephalitis vaccine	تطعيم ضد التهاب الدماغ الياباني
Rh (Anti D) vaccine	تطعيم ضد العامل الرايزسي (مضاد D) في الدم
Meningococcal meningitis vaccine	تطعيم ضد التهاب السحايا بالمكورات السحائية
Tetanus Immunoglobuline	تطعيم خامل ضد الكزاز (التيتانوس)
Human Rotavirus vaccine	تطعيم ضد فيروس الروتا
Anthrax vaccine	تطعيم ضد الجمرة الخبيثة (أنثراكس)
Smallpox vaccine	تعرف على التطعيم ضد الجدري
Cholera Vaccine	تطعيم ضد الكوليرا
Influenza Vaccine H1N1 Swine Flu Vaccine	تطعيم ضد إنفلونزا الخنازير (H1N1)
Pneumococcal conjugate vaccine	لقاح المكورات الرئوية
HPV vaccine	لقاح فيروس الورم الحليمي
Rotavirus vaccine	لقاح الروتا
Varicella virus vaccine	لقاح جدري الماء

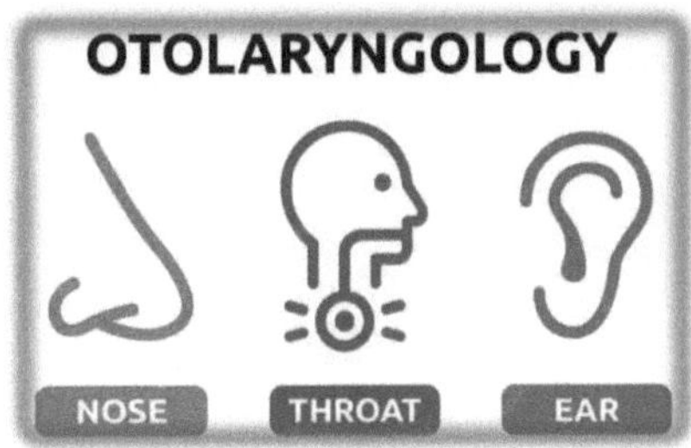

Chapter TWO- Otorhinolaryngology (EAR, NOSE AND THROAT)

Overview

This chapter introduces the reader to common medical terminology of Otorhinolaryngology specialty that will include bilingual terminology for the following;

1. Anatomy
2. Common Symptoms
3. Common Diseases and disorders
4. Further Diseases
5. Investigations
6. Treatments,
7. Surgery and Procedures

We hope you enjoy reading this Chapter, and more chapters awaiting you

- **Anatomy**

ANATOMY OF THE EAR
TEMPORAL MUSCLE
CARTILAGE OF THE AURICLE
TEMPORAL MUSCLE
ABOVE - DRUM RECESS
THE STIRRUP MUSCLE
ABOVE - DRUM RECESS
HAMMER
SEMICIRCULAR CHANNELS
ANVIL
THE AURICLE
NERVE OF THE VESTIBULE
FACIAL NERVE
THE NERVE OF
THE COCHLEA
SNAIL
THE EARDRUM
STIRRUP
ENDOLYMPHOTIC DUCT
EXTERNAL AUDITORY CANAL
ROUND SNAIL WINDOW
THE MUSCLE THAT LIFTS THE PALATINE CURTAIN
THE EUSTACHIAN TUBE
THE MUSCLE STRAINING THE EARDRUM

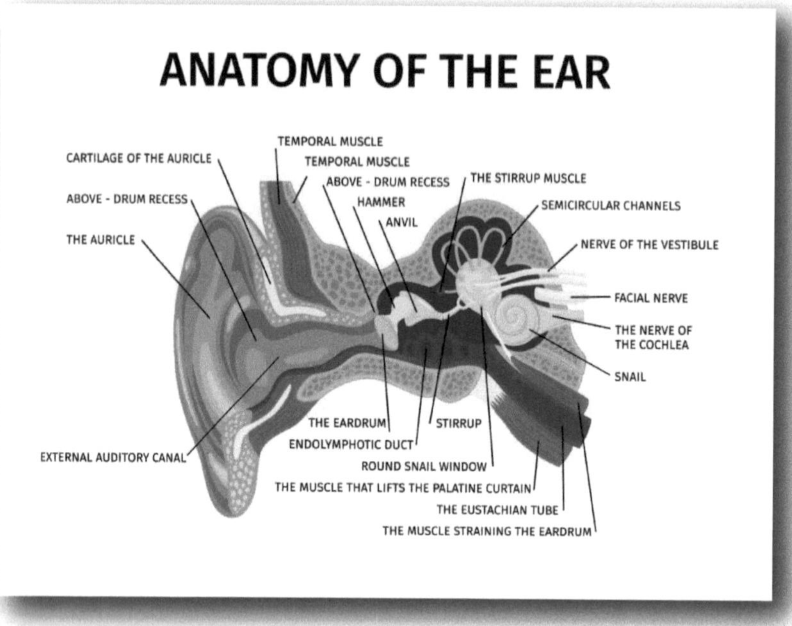

The Common Symptoms	
Term	**المصطلح**
General Symptoms	**أعراض عامة**
Coughing/Sneezing	السعال / العطس
Skin Conditions	الأمراض الجلدية
Skin Cancers/Lesions	سرطانات / آفات الجلد
Pain and pressure	الألم والضغط
Fever	حمى
Nausea and vomiting	غثيان (لوعة) واستفراغ (تقيؤ)
Increased fussiness, especially at bedtime	زيادة الانزعاج ، خاصة في وقت النوم
Eating or drinking abnormally	الأكل أو الشرب بشكل غير طبيعي
Body aches	آلام الجسم
Fatigue	تعب
Headache	صداع
Waking up frequently in the middle of the night	كثرة الاستيقاظ في منتصف الليل
Feeling unrefreshed upon awakening	الشعور بعدم الانتعاش عند الاستيقاظ
Daytime drowsiness	النعاس أثناء النهار
Mood swings	تقلب المزاج
Depression	اكتئاب
Morning headaches	صداع الصباح
Nasal Symptoms (Nose)	**أعراض الآنف**
Sneezing	العطس
Runny Nose (rhinorrhea)	سيلان الأنف (زكام)
Obstructive Sleep Apnea.	توقف التنفس أثناء النوم
Sinus Pressure	ضغط الجيوب الأنفية
Adenoid Inflammation or Infection	التهاب أو عدوى اللحمية
Nose Bleeds	نزيف الأنف
Nasal discharge	بلغم الأنف, مخاط الأنف
Decreased smell	انخفاض في حاسة الشم
Allergy	حساسية
Ear Symptoms	**أعراض الأذن**
Ear Pain.	ألم الأذن
Hearing Loss.	فقدان السمع
Balance Problems	مشاكل التوازن
Ear Noise (Tinnitus) ringing	طنين الأذن
Ear Infection (Otitis Media)	عدوى الأذن (التهاب الأذن الوسطى)
Dizziness	دوخة

Loss of balance	فقدان التوازن
Difficulty hearing	صعوبة في السمع
Fluid discharge (suggestive of a perforation)	افرازات السوائل (يشير إلى وجود ثقب)
Pulling or tugging on the ears	شد أو سحب الأذنين
Failure to startle at loud noises or respond to their name (Absence of Startle reflex – sign of hearing loss in Pediatrics)	عدم التفاعل عند سماع الأصوات العالية أو الضوضاء وعدم الاستجابة على نداء اسماءهم استجابة إجفالية (رد فعل انبهاري)
Ear Discharge	افرازات الأذن
Ear pain	ألم الأذن
Ear wax	شمع الأذن
Ear blockage	انسداد الأذن
Dizziness / Vertigo	الدوخة / الدوار
Throat and Neck Symptoms	**اعراض العنق والحلق**
Snoring.	الشخير
Airway Issues/Difficulty Breathing/Mouth Breathing.	مشاكل مجرى الهواء / صعوبة التنفس / التنفس الفموي
Tonsil Inflammation or Infection	التهاب أو عدوى اللوزتين أو اللحمية
Thyroid Mass	تورم/انتفاخ الغدة الدرقية
Dysphagia (Difficulty Swallowing)	عسر البلع (صعوبة البلع)
Enlarged tonsils	تضخم اللوزتين
Enlarged lymph nodes	تضخم الغدد الليمفاوية
White patches on the tonsils or back of the throat	بقع بيضاء على اللوزتين أو مؤخرة الحلق
Cough	سعال
Congestion	احتقان
Toothache (mainly of the molars)	وجع الأسنان (الأضراس بشكل رئيس)
Waking up with a dry, sore throat	الاستيقاظ مع جفاف الحلق والتهاب
Bad breath (halitosis)	رائحة الفم الكريهة (ظاهرة البخر)
Hemoptysis (the coughing up of blood)	نفث الدم (سعال الدم)

- **The Common Diseases / Health Conditions**

The Common Disease/health conditions	
Term	المصطلح
Nose Disorders	اضطرابات ومشاكل الأنف
Sinusitis	التهابات الجيوب الأنفية
Nasal Polyps	الزوائد الأنفيه -ورم لحمي حميد من الغشاء المخاطي- سليلة)
Allergic Rhinitis	حساسية الأنف
Nasal Septum Deviation	انحراف الحاجز الأنفي
Sleep Apnea	توقف التنفس أثناء النوم
Epistaxis	رعاف (نزيف الأنف)
Anosmia	فقد حاسة الشم
Foreign body	جسم غريب
Ear Disorders	اضطرابات ومشاكل الأذن
Acoustic Neuroma (Vestibular Schwannoma)	ورم العصب السمعي (ورم شفاني الدهليزي)
BPPV: Benign Paroxysmal Positional Vertigo	دوار الوضعي الانتيابي الحميد
Cerumen impaction	انحشار الشمع
Conductive Hearing Loss	فقدان السمع التوصيلي
Ear Drum Perforation	ثقب طبلة الأذن
Facial Nerve Paralysis	شلل العصب الوجهي
Otitis Externa (external ear infection)	التهاب الأذن الخارجية
(Otitis Media) Middle Ear Infection	التهاب الأذن الوسطى
Otosclerosis	تصلب الأذن الوسطى
Sensorineural Hearing Loss (neural hearing loss)	فقدان السمع الحسي العصبي
Tinnitus	طنين الأذن
Perforation of tympanic membrane (eardrum perforation)	انثقاب الغشاء الطبلي
Throat and Neck Disorders	اضطرابات ومشاكل الرقبة والحلق
Pharyngitis	التهابات البلعوم
Laryngitis	التهاب الحنجرة
Epiglottitis	التهاب لسان المزمار
Vocal Cord Nodule	عقيدة الحبل الصوتي
Swollen Lymph nodes	تضخم الغدد الليمفاويه
Upper Respiratory Tract Infection	التهاب الجهاز التنفسي العلوي

Snoring	الشخير
Sleep apnea	توقف التنفس أثناء النوم
Bronchiolitis	التهاب القصيبات الحاد
Tonsillitis	التهاب اللوزتين
Dental infection / caries	تسوس الأسنان

Further Disease/health conditions	
Term	المصطلح
Anosognosia; a condition where you can't recognize other health conditions or problems that you have. Experts commonly describe it as "denial of deficit" or "lack of insight."	عمه العاهة (العجز عن إدراك المرض) حالة لا يمكنك فيها التعرف على الحالات الصحية الأخرى أو المشاكل التي لديك. يصفه الخبراء عادة بأنه "إنكار للعجز" أو "نقص في البصيرة.
congenital malformations	التشوهات الخلقية
Skin Cancer	سرطان الجلد
Ear Disorders	اضطرابات ومشاكل الأذن
Meniere's disease an inner ear problem that can cause dizzy spells, also called vertigo, and hearing loss.	مرض مينير هو اضطراب في الأذن الداخلية يمكن أن يؤدي إلى نوبات دوار (دوار) وفقدان السمع. في معظم الحالات ، يؤثر مرض منيير على أذن واحدة فقط
Autoimmune Inner Ear Disease	أمراض الأذن الداخلية المناعية الذاتية
Bell's Palsy (Facial Nerve Palsy)	شلل بيل أو شلل العصب السابع أو شلل العصب الوجهي
Cholesteatomas an abnormal collection of skin cells deep inside your ear.	وَرَمٌ لُؤْلُؤِي, وَرَمٌ كوليستيرولِيّ
cochlear/acoustic nerve disorders	اضطرابات القوقعة / العصب السمعي
Endolymphatic hydrops = labyrinthine hydrops A disorder of the vestibular system in the inner ear.	زيادة في ضغط سوائل الأذن الداخلية
eustachian tube dysfunction	ضعف قناة استاكيوس
hearing loss	فقدان السمع
hyperacusis (sensitivity to everyday sounds) Super-sensitivity	احتداد السمع (الحساسية للأصوات اليومية)
Labyrinthitis	التهاب تية الأذن (الأذن الداخلية)
otitis externa (swimmer's ear)	التهاب الاذن الخارجية (أذن السباح)
otitis media (chronic ear infection/pain)	التهاب الأذن الوسطى (التهاب الأذن المزمن / الألم)
Otosclerosis	تصلب الأذن الوسطى
Perforated eardrum	ثقب طبلة الأذن
Tinnitus (ringing in the ear)	طنين الأذن (رنين في الأذن)
Vertigo (dizziness)	دوار (دوخة)
Earaches	اوجاع الاذن
Ears and Altitude (Barotrauma) (caused by diving)	إصابة الأذن بالضغط عند الغوص أو التحليق بالجو (بالطائرة)

Earwax (Cerumen Impaction)	انحشار شمع الأذن
Pediatric Hearing Loss	فقدان السمع لدى الأطفال
Ramsay Hunt Syndrome (herpes zoster oticus)	متلازمة رامزي هانت
Nasal Disorders (Nose)	اضطرابات ومشاكل الأنف
Ciliary dysfunction	ضعف الهدبية
sinus disorders	اضطرابات الجيوب الأنفية
submandibular gland for infection or tumor	التهاب أو تورم الغدة تحت الفك السفلي
Deviated Septum	انحراف الحاجز الأنفي
Fungal Sinusitis	التهاب الجيوب الفطري
Geriatric Rhinitis	التهاب الأنف المسن
Nasal Fractures	كسور الأنف
Nasopharyngeal Cancer	سرطان البلعوم الأنفي
Pediatric Sinusitis	التهاب الجيوب عند الأطفال
Pediatric Sleep-disordered Breathing	اضطرابات التنفس أثناء النوم عند الأطفال
Post-nasal Drip	تصريف المخاط عبر الجزء الخلفي من الحلق
Sinus Headaches	صداع الجيوب الأنفية
Sinusitis	التهاب الجيوب الأنفية
Snoring, Sleeping Disorders, and Sleep Apnea	الشخير واضطرابات النوم وتوقف التنفس أثناء النوم
Turbinate Hypertrophy	تضخم التوربينات(قرنية الأنف)
Fracture nasal bone	كسر في عظم الأنف
Nosebleeds (Epistaxis)	نزيف في الأنف
Throat and Neck Disorders	اضطرابات ومشاكل الرقبة والحلق
Tonsil hyperplasia	تضخم اللوزتين
diseases of the parathyroid glands	أمراض الغدد الجار درقية
diseases of the thyroid glands	أمراض الغدد الدرقية
goiter (enlarged thyroid)	دُراق, تضخم الغدة الدرقية (تضخم الدرقية)
Graves' Disease	داء غريفز (الدُّراق الجُحوظيّ)
Hashimoto's Thyroiditis	التهاب الغدة الدرقية هاشيموتو
head and neck cancer	سرطان الرأس والعنق
laryngeal (voice box) tumors	أورام الحنجرة
salivary gland disease	مرض الغدد اللعابية
sensorineural hearing loss	فقدان السمع الحسي العصبي
thyroid cancer	سرطان الغدة الدرقية
thyroid nodules	عقيدات الغدة الدرقية
TMJ (temporomandibular joint / dysfunction)	المفصل الصدغي الفكي (ضعف المفصل الصدغي الفكي)
Tonsillitis	التهاب اللوزتين

vocal cord paralysis	شلل الحبل الصوتي
Aging and Swallowing	الشيخوخة ومشاكل البلع
Ankyloglossia (Tongue-tie)	اللسان المربوط
Asthma	الربو
Bronchitis	التهاب قصبات
Burning Mouth Syndrome	متلازمة حرق الفم
Cleft Lip and Cleft Palate	الشفة الأرنبية وشق سقف الحلق
Conductive Hearing Loss	فقدان السمع التوصيلي
Cricopharyngeal Muscle Dysfunction	ضعف العضلات الحلقية
Dry Mouth Syndrome	متلازمة جفاف الفم
Dysgeusia	عسر (خلل) الذوق
GERD and LPR gastroesophageal reflux disease (GERD) laryngopharyngeal reflux (LPR)	ارتجاع المريء المعدي وارتجاع الحنجري البلعومي
Head and Neck Cancer	سرطان الرأس والرقبة
Human Papillomavirus (HPV)	فيروس الورم الحليمي البشري(HPV)
Hoarseness	بحة في الصوت
Hyperthyroidism	فرط نشاط الغدة الدرقية
Hyposmia and Anosmia	نقص حاسة الشم وفقدان الشم
Neck Mass in Adults	كتلة العنق عند البالغين
Oral Lichen Planus	الحزاز المسطح الفموي
Otosclerosis	تصلب الأذن
Pediatric Gastroesophageal Reflux Disease (GERD)	ارتجاع المريء المعدي لدى الأطفال (جيرد)
Pediatric Thyroid Cancer	سرطان الغدة الدرقية لدى الأطفال
Recurrent Respiratory Papillomatosis (RRP)	الورم الحليمي التنفسي المتكرر (RRP)
Rhinitis	التهاب الأنف
Salivary Gland Disorders	اضطرابات الغدد اللعابية
Sensorineural Hearing Loss (SNHL)	فقدان السمع الحسي العصبي (SNHL)
Sialadenitis	التهاب الغدد اللعابية
Sore Throats	التهاب الحلق
Spasmodic Dysphonia	خلل النطق التشنجي
Temporo-Mandibular Joint (TMJ) Pain	آلام مفصل الفك الصدغي (TMJ)
Thyroid Cancer	سرطان الغدة الدرقية
Thyroid Nodules	عقيدات الغدة الدرقية
Tonsillitis	التهاب اللوزتين
Tonsils and Adenoids	اللوزتين واللحمية

Vestibular Schwannoma (Acoustic Neuroma)	الورم الشفاني الدهليزي (الورم العصبي السمعي)
Voice Box (Laryngeal) Cancer	سرطان الحنجرة (الأحبال الصوتية)
Zenker's Diverticulum	رتج زنكر

- Investigations

Investigations	
Diagnostic Service	المصطلح
Laboratory	فحوصات المختبر (المعمل)
CBC – Complete Blood Count (FBC – Full Blood Count)	تحليل تعداد الدم الكامل
Allergy skin test	اختبار حساسية الجلد
Immunoglobulin estimate	تقدير الغلوبولين المناعي
Bleeding disorder test	اختبار اضطراب النزيف
Activated Partial Thromboplastin Time	اختبار زمن الترمبوبلاستين الجزئي
Prothrombin Time	
International Normalized Ratio (INR)	
Thyroid function test	فحص الغدة الدرقية
Fine needle aspiration (FNA)	الشفط بالإبرة الدقيقة (FNA)
Radiology	فحوصات الأشعة التصويرية
X-ray sinuses	تصوير الجيوب الأنفية بالأشعة السينية
X-ray Nasal bone	تصوير بالأشعة السينية لعظم الأنف
X-ray soft tissue (lateral neck)	تصوير بالأشعة السينية للأنسجة الرخوة (الرقبة للجانبين)
X-ray mastoid (ears)	الأشعة السينية لعظمة خشاء الأذن
MRI Mead	التصوير بالرنين المغناطيسي للرأس
CT (Head)	تصوير مقطعي للرأس
CT (para-nasal-sinus)	التصوير المقطعي المحوسب (الأنف والجيوب الأنفية)
CT (Ears)	التصوير المقطعي (آذان)
CT (Neck)	التصوير المقطعي (الرقبة)
Ultrasound Neck	الموجات فوق الصوتية للرقبة
Hearing test	فحص السمع
Pure Tone Audiometry	قياس السمع
Tympanometry And Reflex	فحص ضغط الأذن
Eviked Otoacoustic Emissions	الانبعاث القوقعي
Conditioning Play Audiometry	قياس سمع الأطفال
VRA Test	قياس سمع الأطفال بالتعزيز المرئي
Auditory Evoked Potentials	استجابة جذع الدماغ
Balance test	فحص التوازن

CVEMP test	فحص استجابة التوازن
ECOG test	تخطيط كهربائية القوقعة
Hearing aid check	فحص السماعة
Basic vestibular evaluation	فحص التوازن الأساسي
Caloric vestibular test	فحص التوازن بالماء
Rotary chair assessment	فحص الكرسي الدوار
CDP test	فحص ثبات التوازن
Dix-hallpike maneuver	تمارين التوازن ديكس هولبيك
Epley maneuver	تمارين التوازن ايبلي

- ## Treatment

Treatment	
Term	المصطلح
Medications	أدوية
Antibiotic medicine	المضادات الحيوية
Pain killer medicine	مسكن للألم
Antihistamine medicine	مضادات الهيستامين
Anti-vertigo medicine	المضادات للدوار
Anti-acidity medicine	المضادات للحموضة
Nasal spray (steroid, saline, decongestant)	بخاخ للأنف (كورتيزون ، محلول ملحي ، مزيل للاحتقان)
Ear drop	قطرة الأذن
Gargles	الغرغرة
Ointment	مرهم
Aerosol and humidity therapy– CPT, postural drainage and percussion	العلاج باستنشاق البخار والرطوبة – العلاج الطبيعي للصدر والنزح الوضعي والنقر
(respiratory physiotherapy) (nebulizer)	(العلاج الطبيعي للجهاز التنفسي)
audiology/hearing aids	السمع / السماعات الطبية
Speech therapy	جلسات لعلاج أمراض النطق واللغة
Surgery / procedure	جراحة / إجراءات طبية

Surgery / Procedures	
Term	المصطلح
Ear Surgery	جراحة الأذن
Myringotomy with grommet insertion(for middle ear fluid) Surgical incision into the eardrum, to relieve pressure or drain fluid.	عمل بضع لطبلة الأذن مع ادخال أنبوب شق جراحي في طبلة الأذن لتخفيف الضغط أو تصريف السوائل.
Tympanostomy tubes will be placed to allow fluid to pass through the ear canal into the middle ear.	فغر الطبلة وتركيب أنبوب سيتم وضع الأنابيب للسماح للسوائل بالمرور عبر قناة الأذن إلى الأذن الوسطى.
cochlear implants The implant has external and internal parts. The external part sits behind the ear. It picks up sounds with a microphone. It then processes the sound and transmits it to the internal part of the implant.	زراعة قوقعة الأذن يحتوي الزرع على أجزاء خارجية وداخلية. الجزء الخارجي خلف الأذن. يلتقط الأصوات بالميكروفون. ثم تقوم بمعالجة الصوت ونقله إلى الجزء الداخلي من الغرسة.
Nasal Surgery (Nose)	جراحة الأنف
Septoplasty is a surgical procedure to straighten the bone and cartilage dividing the space between your two nostrils (septum). When the septum is crooked, it is known as a deviated septum.	رأب الحاجز الأنفي هو إجراء جراحي لتقويم العظام والغضاريف وتقسيم المسافة بين فتحتي الأنف (الحاجز). عندما يكون الحاجز معوجًا ، يُعرف باسم الحاجز المنحرف.
Septorhinoplasty (Rhoinoplasty) is an operation to improve the appearance of your nose (rhinoplasty) and to improve how you breathe through your nose (septoplasty). It involves operating on the bones and cartilage that give your nose its shape and structure and making your septum straight.	تجميل الأنف هي عملية لتحسين مظهر أنفك (تجميل الأنف) ولتحسين طريقة تنفسك من خلال أنفك (رأب الحاجز الأنفي). إنه ينطوي على إجراء عملية على العظام والغضاريف التي تعطي أنفك شكلها وهيكلها وتجعل حاجزك مستقيماً.
Turbinectomy 'is a procedure in which some or all of the turbinate bones in the nasal passage are removed, generally to relieve nasal obstruction. In most cases, turbinate hypertrophy is accompanied by some septum deviation, so the surgery is done along with septoplasty.	استئصال قرنية الأنف هو إجراء يتم فيه إزالة بعض أو كل عظام المحارة في الممر الأنفي ، بشكل عام لتخفيف انسداد الأنف. في معظم الحالات ، يكون تضخم المحارة مصحوبًا ببعض انحراف الحاجز ، لذلك تتم الجراحة جنبًا إلى جنب مع رأب الحاجز الأنفي.
Adenoidectomy	استئصال لحمية الأنف
Throat and Neck Surgery	جراحة الرقبة والحلق
Tonsillectomy	إستئصال اللوزتين
Tonsillectomy (ton-sih-LEK-tuh-me) is the surgical removal of the tonsils, two oval-shaped pads of tissue at the back of the throat — one tonsil on each side.	استئصال اللوزتين (ton-sih-LEK-tuh-me) هو الاستئصال الجراحي للوزتين ، وهما وسادتان بيضاويتان من الأنسجة في مؤخرة الحلق ـ لوزة واحدة على كل جانب.

Tonsillotomy	بضع اللوزتين
partial removal of the tonsils	استئصال جزئي للوزتين
Parathyroidectomy	استئصال جارات الغدة الدرقية
Thyroidectomy	استئصال الغدة الدرقية
Parotidectomy	استئصال الغدة النكفية
Foreign body removal	إزالة جسم غريب

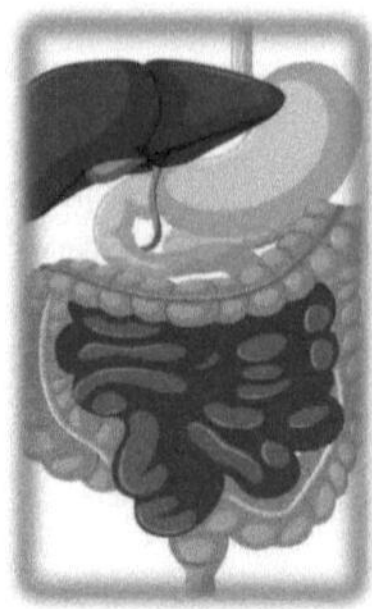

Chapter THREE – Gastroenterology

Overview

This chapter introduces the reader to common medical terminology of Gastroenterology specialty that will include bilingual terminology for the following;

1. Anatomy
2. Common Symptoms
3. Main Common Diseases / Health Conditions
4. Investigations
5. Treatments
6. Surgery / Procedure
7. Complications

We hope you enjoy reading this Chapter, and more chapters awaiting you

INTERNAL HUMAN
DIGESTIVE SYSTEM

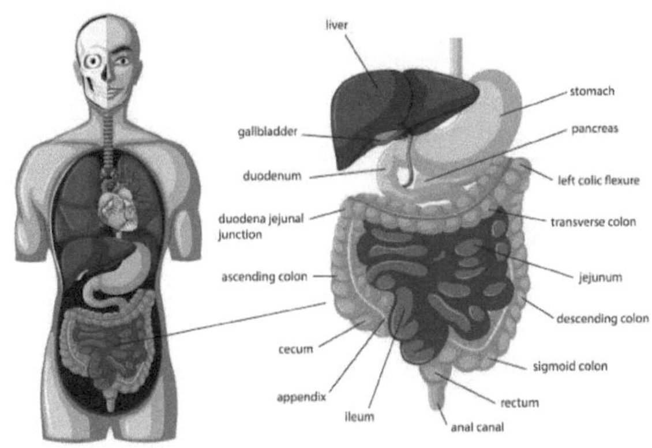

DIGESTION PROCESS

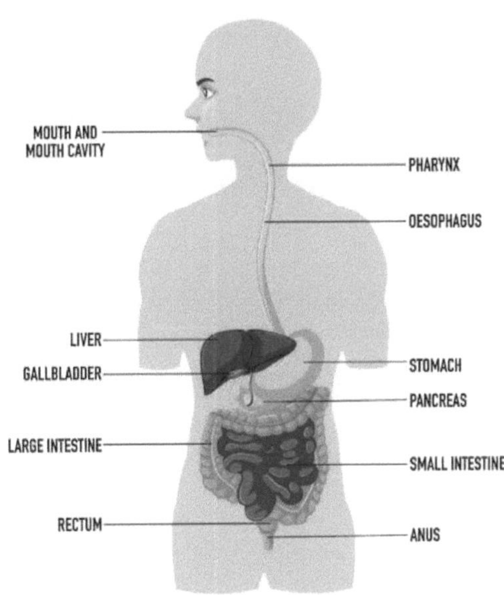

- **The Common Symptoms**

The Common Symptoms	
Term **General Symptoms**	المصطلح أعراض عامة
Abdominal discomfort	عدم ارتياح في البطن
pain or cramps	ألم وتقلصات (مغص معوي)
Unintentional weight loss	فقدان (خسارة) الوزن الغير متعمد
Vomiting and nausea	القيء والغثيان
Acid reflux (heartburn)	الارتجاع الحمضي (حرقة المعدة) – صاهر
Diarrhea	الإسهال
Constipation	الإمساك
Nausea	الغثيان (اللوعة)
Vomiting (throwing up)	التقيؤ
Vomiting blood or darker fluids that appear like coffee grounds (Hematemesis)	تقيؤ الدم أو السوائل الداكنة التي تبدو مثل القهوة المطحونة
Bloating	انتفاخ
Fecal incontinence	سلس البراز (تبرز لا إرادي)، عدم السيطرة على البراز
Fatigue/tiredness	تعب شديد / إرهاق
Loss of appetite	فقدان الشهية
Difficulty swallowing.	صعوبة في الابتلاع
Bleeding in the digestive tract.	نزيف في الجهاز الهضمي.
Severe and persistent indigestion.	عسر الهضم الشديد والمستمر.
Stomach upset	اضطراب المعدة.
Ulcers.	قرحة.
Excess gas.	الغازات الزائدة.
Change in bowel habits such as harder, looser, or more urgent stools than normal.	تغير في عادات الأمعاء مثل البراز الأكثر صلابة أو الليونة أو المستعجلة أكثر من المعتاد.
Alternating constipation and diarrhea.	تناوب الإمساك والإسهال.
Blood on or in the stool that is either bright or dark red.	دم في البراز يكون أحمر ناصع أو داكن.
Unusual abdominal or gas pains.	آلام غير عادية في البطن أو الغازات.
Very narrow stool.	براز رفيع جدا.
A feeling that the bowel has not emptied completely after passing stool.	شعور بعدم إفراغ الأمعاء تمامًا بعد خروج البراز.
Anemia (low blood count).	فقر الدم (انخفاض نسبة الدم).
Chest or abdominal pain	ألم في الصدر أو البطن
Black or bloody bowel movements	حركات الأمعاء مع لون براز أحمر أو داكن

Severe headache	صداع حاد
Stiff neck	تصلب الرقبة
A fever higher than 101 °F	حمى أعلى من 101 درجة فهرنهايت
Exhaustion or trouble waking up	الإرهاق أو صعوبة الاستيقاظ
Dehydration symptoms including feeling tired, a high degree of thirst, dry mouth, muscle cramps, dizziness, confusion, dark colored urine or a lack of the need to urinate	أعراض الجفاف بما في ذلك الشعور بالتعب ، ودرجة عالية من العطش ، وجفاف الفم ، وتشنجات العضلات ، والدوخة ، والارتباك ، والبول داكن اللون أو عدم الحاجة إلى التبول
Burping	التجشؤ
can't digest fatty foods	لا يستطيع هضم الأطعمة الدهنية
diarrhea after meals	الإسهال بعد الوجبات
Gallstones	حصى المرارة
liver disease	مرض الكبد
pancreas inflammation	التهاب البنكرياس
inflammation of stomach and intestines	التهاب المعدة والأمعاء
gallbladder inflammation	التهاب المرارة
scarring of the liver	تليف الكبد
stomach pain upper left side	آلام المعدة في الجانب الأيسر العلوي
stomach pain upper right side	آلام المعدة في الجانب الأيمن العلوي
stomach pain lower left side	آلام في المعدة أسفل الجانب الأيسر
stomach pain lower right side	آلام في المعدة أسفل الجانب الأيمن
lower stomach pain	آلام أسفل المعدة
pain near belly button spreading to lower right side of stomach	ينتشر الألم بالقرب من السرة إلى الجانب الأيمن السفلي من المعدة
upper stomach pain	آلام في الجزء العلوي من المعدة
ulcer in area connecting stomach to duodenum	قرحة في المنطقة التي تربط المعدة بالاثني عشر
upper belly bloating	انتفاخ الجزء العلوي من البطن
bladder distention	امتلاء المثانة
bladder feels full	يشعر المثانة بالامتلاء
epigastric abdominal tenderness	إيلام (احساس بالألم مع اللمس) البطن الشرسوفي
feels like need to pee all the time	أشعر بالحاجة إلى التبول طوال الوقت
lower belly bloating	انتفاخ أسفل البطن

- ## The Common Diseases / Health Conditions

The Common Disease/health conditions	
Term	**المصطلح**
Irritable Bowel Syndrome (IBS)	متلازمة القولون العصبي(IBS)
Inflammatory bowel disease (IBD)	
Inflammatory bowel disease (Crohn's disease and ulcerative colitis)	مرض التهاب الأمعاء (مرض كرون والتهاب القولون التقرحي)
Celiac Disease	الداء الزلاقي (الداء البطني) الحساسية من الجلوتين (القمح)
Bowel Control Problems (Fecal Incontinence)	مشاكل التحكم في الأمعاء (سلس البراز)
flatulence (Gas)	غازات
Lactose Intolerance	عدم تحمل(حساسية) من اللاكتوز
Diarrhea	إسهال
Constipation	إمساك
Chronic Diarrhea	الإسهال المزمن
Heartburn	حرقة في المعدة
Stomach problems	مشاكل في المعدة
Acid Reflux (GER & GERD)	الارتجاع الحمضي(GER & GERD)
Chronic Diarrhea in Children	الإسهال المزمن عند الأطفال
Constipation in Children	الإمساك عند الأطفال
Hirschsprung Disease	مرض هيرشسبرونج
Irritable Bowel Syndrome (IBS) in Children	متلازمة القولون العصبي (IBS) عند الأطفال
Abdominal Adhesions	التصاقات البطن
Anatomic Problems of the Lower GI Tract	المشاكل التشريحية للجهاز الهضمي السفلي
Appendicitis	التهاب الزائدة الدودية
Barrett's Esophagus	مرض المريء نوع باريت
Colon Polyps	الأورام الحميدة في القولون – لحميات القولون
Cyclic Vomiting Syndrome	متلازمة التقيؤ الدوري
Dumping Syndrome (Rapid gastric emptying)	متلازمة الإغراق (الإفراغ السريع للمعدة)
a group of symptoms, such as diarrhea, nausea, and feeling light-headed or tired after a meal, that are caused by rapid gastric emptying	وهي مجموعة من الأعراض ، مثل الإسهال والغثيان والشعور بالدوخة أو التعب بعد الأكل ، والتي تنتج عن إفراغ المعدة السريع.

Exocrine Pancreatic Insufficiency (EPI)	قصور البنكرياس الإفرازي (EPI)
Food Poisoning (foodborne illness)	تسمم غذائي (المرض المنقول عن طريق الغذاء)
Gallstones	حصى المرارة
Gastritis	التهاب المعدة
Microscopic Colitis	التهاب القولون المجهري
Pancreatitis	التهاب البنكرياس
Proctitis	التهاب المستقيم
Ulcerative Colitis	التهاب القولون التقرحي
Viral Gastroenteritis	التهاب المعدة والأمعاء الفيروسي
Diverticulosis & Diverticulitis	الرتج والتهاب الرتج
Colitis	التهاب القولون
Acute and Chronic Pancreatitis	التهاب البنكرياس الحاد والمزمن
Gastroparesis (paralysis of the stomach)	خزل المعدة
GI Bleeding	نزيف الجهاز الهضمي
Hemorrhoids	بواسير
Indigestion (Dyspepsia)	عسر الهضم (عسر الهضم)
Inguinal Hernia	الفتق الإربي
Intestinal Pseudo-obstruction	انسداد الأمعاء الزائف
Liver Disease	مرض الكبد
Peptic Ulcers (Stomach Ulcers)	القرحة الهضمية (قرحة المعدة)
Short Bowel Syndrome	متلازمة الأمعاء القصيرة
Zollinger-Ellison Syndrome	متلازمة زولينجر إليسون
H. pylori (Helicobacter pylori)	جرثومة المعدة
Esophagitis is inflammation of the esophagus	التهاب المريء

- **Investigations**

Investigations	
Diagnostic Service	المصطلح
Laboratory	فحوصات المختبر (المعمل)
Blood test	فحص الدم
Stool test	اختبار البراز
Urine test	فحص بول
Breath test	اختبار التنفس
Polyps biopsy test	اختبار خزعة الزوائد اللحمية
Radiology	الأشعة التشخيصية
DEXA scan; measure bone density (thickness and strength of bones)	فحص هشاشة العظام، مسح DEXA قياس كثافة العظام (سمك وقوة العظام)
Ultrasound	الموجات فوق الصوتية
MRI	التصوير بالرنين المغناطيسي
CT Scan	الاشعة المقطعية
esophagogram (Barium swallow), is an imaging test that checks for problems in your upper GI tract.	اشعة المرئ الملونة بالباريوم، هو اختبار تصوير يتحقق من وجود مشاكل في الجهاز الهضمي العلوي.
Endoscopy Procedures	المناظير
Endoscopic ultrasound (EUS)	الموجات فوق الصوتية بالمنظار (EUS)
Endoscopic retrograde cholangiopancreatography (ERCP)	تصوير البنكرياس والقنوات الصفراوية بالمنظار (ERCP)
Endoscopic mucosal resection (EMR)	استئصال الغشاء المخاطي بالمنظار (EMR)
PEG (percutaneous endoscopic gastrostomy)	فتح المعدة بالمنظار عن طريق الجلد PEG
a procedure in which a flexible feeding tube is placed through the abdominal wall and into the stomach.	إجراء يتم فيه وضع أنبوب تغذية مرن عبر جدار البطن وصولاً إلى المعدة.
Colonoscopy	تنظير القولون
Procedure	الإجراءات الطبية
Upper GI Endoscopy, EGD (esophagogastroduodenoscopy) is a procedure to diagnose and treat problems in your upper GI (gastrointestinal) tract	تنظير المريء والمعدة والأمعاء EGD هو إجراء لتشخيص وعلاج المشاكل في الجزء الأعلى من الجهاز الهضمي
Colonoscopy	منظار القولون
Endoscopic retrograde cholangio pancreatography (ERCP)	تصوير البنكرياس الصفراوي الوراثي بالمنظار(ERCP)
Flexible Sigmoidoscopy	تنظير القولون السيني
Virtual Colonoscopy	تنظير القولون الافتراضي
Breath Test / Urea Breath Test (UBT)	اختبار التنفس / اختبار التنفس اليوريا (UBT)

For H. Pylori (Helicobacter Pylori)	لجرثومة الملوية البوابية (هيليكوباكتر بيلوري)
The glucose tolerance test (OGTT-Oral Glucose Challenge Test) is given to determine how quickly glucose is cleared from the blood.	اختبار تحمل الجلوكوز (اختبار تحدي الجلوكوز الفموي OGTT) يتم الاختبار لتحديد مدى سرعة إزالة الجلوكوز من الدم.
A Fructose Intolerance Test shows how you digest certain carbohydrates or sugars, e.g. lactose or fruit sugar, called 'fructose'.	اختبار عدم تحمل الفركتوز، يوضح كيف يمكنك هضم بعض الكربوهيدرات أو السكريات ، على سبيل المثال اللاكتوز أو سكر الفاكهة ، ويسمى "الفركتوز".
A lactose tolerance test measures how well your body can process lactose, a type of sugar found in dairy products.	اختبار تحمل اللاكتوز، يقيس مدى قدرة جسمك على هضم اللاكتوز ، وهو نوع من السكر الموجود في مشتقات الحليب.

- Treatment

Treatment	
Term	المصطلح
Medications	أدوية
Antibiotic medicine	المضادات الحيوية
Analgesics (Pain killer)	مسكن ألم
Antacids	مضادات الحموضة
Antidiarrheals	مضادات الإسهال
Antiemetics	مضادات القيء
Antifungals	مضادات الفطريات
Antihistamines	مضادات الهيستامين (للحساسية)
Antipyretics	خافضات الحرارة
Antivirals	مضادات الفيروسات
Diuretics	مدرات البول
IV injections	حقن وريدية
Syrup for bloating, gases and acidity	شراب للانتفاخات والغازات والحموضة
Cream for hemorrhoids	كريم للبواسير
Suppository	تحميلة

- ## Surgery / Procedures

Term	المصطلح
Gastroscopy	تنظير المعدة
Colonscopy	تنظير القولون
Endoscopic retrograde cholangiopancreatography (ERCP)	تصوير البنكرياس والقنوات الصفراوية بالمنظار (ERCP)
PH manometry	قياس الأس الهيدروجيني
Colorectal surgery	جراحة القولون والمستقيم
Polyp removal	إزالة الزوائد اللحمية
Dilation of the esophagus with the stent	توسيع المريء بالدعامة
Ostomy Surgery of the Bowel	جراحة فغر الأمعاء

- ## Complications

Term	المصطلح
Allergic reaction to the medicine	رد فعل تحسسي للدواء
Infection	عدوى
Bleeding	نزيف
Recurrence of the polyps and the hemorrhoids	معاودة ظهور الأورام الحميدة والبواسير
Perforation	انثقاب
Recurrence of H. Pylori	تكرار الإصابة بالبكتيريا الحلزونية البوابية
Reaction to sedation or anesthesia	رد فعل للتنويم أو التخدير
Fever	حمى
Chest pain	ألم صدر
Shortness of breath	ضيق في التنفس
Difficulty in swallowing (dysphagia)	صعوبة في البلع (عسر البلع)
Vomiting	التقيؤ
Abdominal pain	وجع بطن
Colorectal surgery	جراحة القولون والمستقيم
Polyp removal	إزالة الزوائد اللحمية

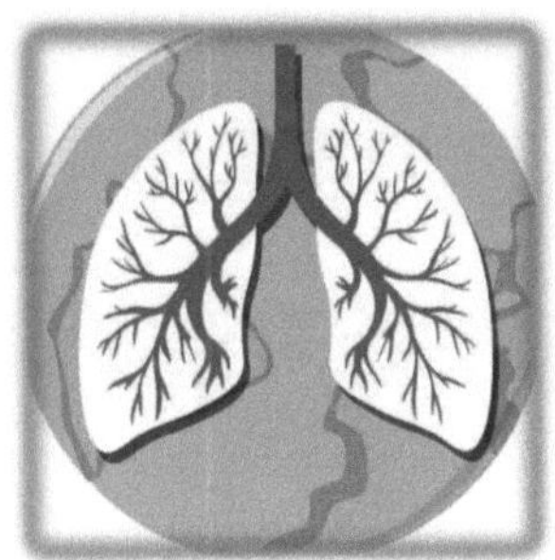

Chapter FOUR – Pulmonology

Overview

This chapter introduces the reader to common medical terminology of Pulmonology that will include bilingual terminology for the following;

1. Anatomy
2. Common Symptoms
3. Main Common Diseases / Health Conditions
4. Further Diseases / Health Conditions
5. Investigations
6. Skin Prick test
7. Treatments

We hope you enjoy reading this Chapter, and more chapters awaiting you

- ## Anatomy

Trachea
Apex
Right upper lobe
Left upper lobe
Right bronchus
Hilum
Left bronchus
Horizontal fissure
Right middle lobe
Bronchioles
Oblique fissure
Right lower lobe
Left lower lobe
Cardiac notch
Base of lung

Superior Horn of thyroid Cartilage
Left lamina of thyroid Cartilage
Right lamina of thyroid Cartilage
Thyroid Cartilage
Median cricothyroid ligament
Cricoid Cartilage
Upper lobe
Trachel cartilages
Right bronchus
Mucosa of posterior tracheal wall
Bronchus lobaris superior dexter
Anular ligaments
Bronchus intermediale
Trachea
Bronchus lobaris medius dexter
Tracheal bifurcation
Horizontal fissure
Left bronchus
Middle lobe
Oblique fissure
Bronchus lobaris inferior dexter
Upper lobe
Oblique fissure
Lower lobe
Lower lobe
Notch for the heart
Right lobe
Left lobe

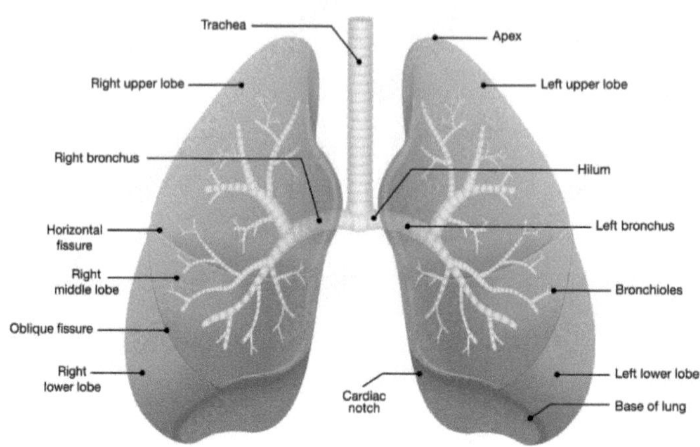

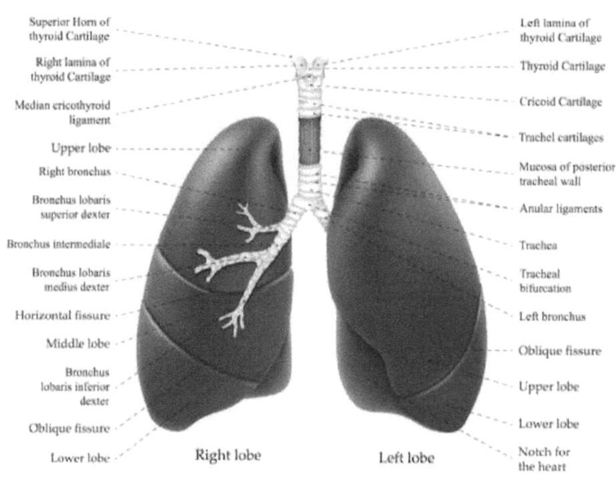

Respiratory system

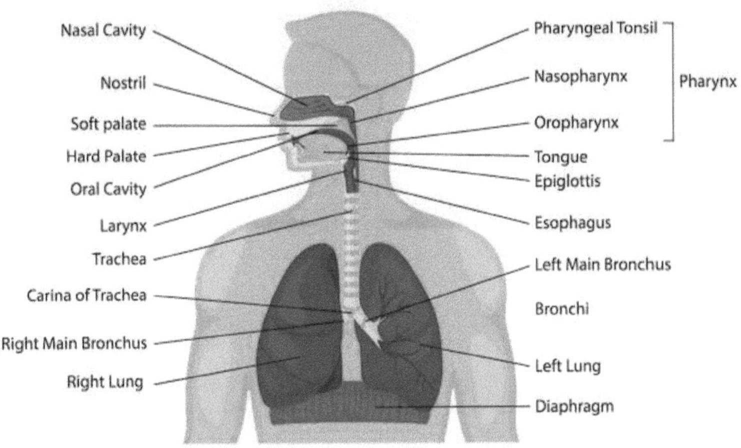

The Common Symptoms	
Term	المصطلح
Sneezing	العطس
Snoring	الشخير
Cough	سعال، كحة
Runny nose (rhinorrhea)	رشح (سيلان الأنف) سيلان الأنف
Blocked nose (stuffy nose), Nasal congestion	انسداد الأنف (انسداد الأنف)، احتقان في الأنف
Foul smell, bad smelling, malodorous smell	رائحة كريهة
Nausea(sickness)	غثيان، لوعة
Vomiting (emesis)	التقيؤ
Fever (pyrexia)	حمى
Apnea	انقطاع النفس
Throat dryness (xerostomia)	جفاف الحلق
Dyspnoea (shortness of breath)	ضيق التنفس
Dysphonia (hoarseness of voice)	بحة الصوت
Chest pain	ألم في الصدر
Chest Tightness	ضيق في الصدر
Chest distress	ضيق في الصدر، ثقل على الصدر
Wheezing	صفير، أزيز
Fatigue	تعب
Headache	صداع
Back pain	ألم في الظهر
Shoulder pain	الم الكتف
Abdominal pain	وجع بطن
(visceral pain or peritoneal pain)	(ألم حشوي، صفاقي)
Weight loss	فقدان الوزن
Acid reflux, GERD (gastroesophagial reflux disease)	ارتجاع حمضي
Sleep symptoms	أعراض النوم
Tiredness	التعب، الإرهاق
Sleepiness	النعاس
Distracted sleep	النوم المشتت
Difficulty to initiate sleep	صعوبة بدء النوم
Restless legs	تململ الساقين، متلازمة الساق القلقة
Abnormal sleep behavioral (walking,	سلوكات أثناء النوم غير طبيعية (مشي، تحدث، كوابيس)

Term	المصطلح
talking, acting dreams)	
Stomach bloating (from CPAP)	انتفاخات المعدة بسبب CPAP
Sleep paralysis	شلل النوم
Narcolepsy	النوم القهري – النوم بشكل مفاجئ
Insomnia, Sleeplessness	أرق
Cataplexy	الجمدة
Rapid or irregular heartbeat.	سرعة ضربات القلب أو عدم انتظامها.
Light headedness or dizziness.	الدوار أو الدوخة.
Excessive sweating.	التعرق المفرط.
Cyanosis (a bluish-purple hue to the skin.)	الإزرقاق، الزراق
Haemoptysis (coughing up blood)	نفث الدم، سعال الدم
Expectoration (spitting out sputum)	نخامة، طرد البلغم
Palpitation (A rapid or irregular heartbeat)	خفقان
Hallucination , delirium	الهلوسة، هذيان

- ## The Common Diseases / Health Conditions

The Common Disease/health conditions	
Term	المصطلح
Bronchial Asthma	الربو الشعبي
Chronic Obstructive Pulmonary Disease (COPD)	مرض انسداد القصبات الرئوي المزمن
Emphysema	انتفاخ الرئة
Chest Infection	التهاب الصدر
Pneumonia	الالتهاب الرئوي (ذات الرئة)
Bronchitis	التهاب الشعب الهوائية / التهاب القصبات الهوائية
Sleep Apnea Syndrome	متلازمة انقطاع التنفس أثناء النوم
Pulmonary Vascular Disease	أمراض الأوعية الدموية الرئوية
Pleural Disease	الأنصباب الجنبي
Pulmonary Fibrosis	التليف الرئوي
Upper Airways Disease	مرض مجرى الهواء العلوي
Lung Cancer	سرطان الرئة
Chest Wall Disease	أمراض القفص الصدري
Asthma	ربو
Cystic fibrosis	التليف الكيسي الرئوي

Pulmonary edema	وذمه رئوية
Pulmonary embolism	الانسداد الرئوي (الجلطة الرئوية)
Tuberculosis	مرض السل (الدرن)
Allergies;	**الحساسية:**
Pollen, molds, animal dander, latex, certain foods and insect stings.	حبيبات اللقاح، العفن, وبر الحيوانات, المطاط, بعض أنواع الأطعمة, السم من جراء لسعة النحل
Croup	الخانوق
Cyanosis	الزراق
Bronchiolitis	التهاب القصيبات
Respiratory syncytial virus - RSV	الفيروس المخلوي التنفسي
Bronchiectasis	توسع القصبات
Chronic Cough	السعال المزمن
Common cold	الزكام
Upper Respiratory Tract Infection	التهابات المجاري التنفسية العليا
Sore Throat	التهاب الحلق
Restless leg syndrome (jimmy leg – Von Ekbom's syndrome)	متلازمة تململ الساقين ، الساق القلقة، اهتزاز الساق، متلازمة ايبكوم
Pleural effusion	الانصبابُ الجنبي (تراكم السوائل في بطانة الرئة)
Empyema (puss in the pleural cavity)	تجمع قيحي بالغشاء الجنبي (خراج الغشاء الجنبي)
Dysfunctional breathing	اختلال في عملية التنفس (التنفس بشكل سريع)
Diaphragmatic palsy	شلل الحجاب الحاجز

- **Further Diseases / Health Conditions**

Further Disease/health conditions	
Term	المصطلح
Granuloma	الورم الحبيبي
Interstitial lung disease	مرض رئوي خلالي (أمراض تليف الرئة)
Nodule	عقدة
Pneumoconiosis	تغبر الرئة
Pulmonary hypertension	ارتفاع ضغط الدم بالشريان الرئوي
Respiratory failure	قصور الجهاز التنفسي
Sarcoidosis	الساركويد
Trachea stenosis	تضيق القصبة الهوائية
Lung air leak	تسرب الهواء من الرئة
Lung abscess	خراج الرئة
Lung - congenital defects	ـ عيوب الرئة الخلقية
Laryngitis: acute/chronic	ـالتهاب الحنجرة
Psittacosis	الببغائية
Pertusis	الشاهوق
(Bordetella Pertussis)	(جرثومة البروديتيلة الشاهوقية)
Respiratory insufficiency	الفشل التنفسي
Hypoxia	نقص التأكسج (الأكسجين)
ARDS- Acute respiratory distress syndrome	متلازمة الفشل التنفسي الحاد
Bacterial pneumonia	التهاب رئوي جرثومي
Sleep apnea syndrome	متلازمة انقطاع النفس النومي
Bronchopleural fistula	الناسور القصبي الجنبي
Congenital deformities of the chest wall	تشوهات خلقية في جدار الصدر
Funnel chest (= pectus excavatum)	صدر مقعر
Pigeon breast (= pectus carinatum)	صدر جؤجؤي – صدر دجاجة
Bronchogenic cyst	كيسة قصبية المنشأ
Middle lobe syndrome	متلازمة الفص المتوسط
Abdominal wall congenital malformations	تشوهات خلقية في جدار البطن
Embryogenesis	عملية تطور الجنين (التخلق)
Mediastinitis	التهاب المنصف
Pancoast tumor	ورم بانكوست
Lung contusion	الكدمة الرئوية
Flail chest	الصدر السائب
Chylothorax	الكيلوس في الصدر
Pneumothorax	الاسترواح الصدري (الهواء في غشاء الجنب)

Empyema	دبيلة (تجمع قيحي في غشاء الجنب)
Bulla	الفقاعات
Blebectomy	استئصال الفقاعات الصدرية
Lung hernia	فتق الرئة
Tumors of trachea	أورام الرغامى
Benign tumors of the lung	أورام حميدة في الرئة
Hemothorax	انصباب جنبي دموي وهوائي
Stridor	صرير
Pulmonary sequestration	الانحجازُ الرئوي (انحباس جزء من الرئة)
Pneumocystis Carinii Pneumonia	التهاب رئوي بالمتكيسة الجؤجؤية
Yellow nail syndrome	متلازمة الظفر الأصفر
Chronic-Obstructive Pulmonary Disease	مرض الانسداد الرئوي المزمن
Interstitial lung disease	الأمراض الخلالية الرئوية
Respiratory muscles diseases	أمراض عضلات الجهاز التنفسي
Adenosine deaminase deficiency	نقص إنزيم الـ أدينوسين دي أمينيز
Goodpasture's Syndrome	متلازمة غود باستشار
Mitochondrial respiratory chain defects	امراض السلسلة التنفسية الميتوكوندريا
Congenital anomalies of the airways	تشوهات خلقية في ممرات الهواء
Recurrent and persistent cough	السعال عند الاطفال
Croup	الخانوق
Restrictive lung disease	أمراض الرئة المقيدة (المُحِددة)
Asphyxia of newborn	اختناق الوليد
Bronchopulmonary dysplasia	خلل التنسج القصبي الرئوي
Sputum	البلغم
Bronchiolitis	التهاب القصيبات
Recurrent pneumonia in children	الالتهاب الرئوي عند الاطفال
Productive cough	السعال
Bronchiectasis	توسع القصبات
Berylliosis	التسمم بالبريليوم
Eosinophilic pneumonia	الالتهاب الرئوي اليوزيني
Anthrax	الجمرة الخبيثة
Asbestosis	داء الأسبست
Byssinosis	السحارُ القطني
Silicosis	السحار السيليسي
Mushroom worker's lungs, Extrinsic allergic alveolitis (Hypersensitivity pneumonitis).	تلوث رئوي من فطريات التهاب فطري رئوي بفرط التحسس

Thoracic outlet syndrome - TOS	متلازمة مخرج الصدر
Guillain-Barre Syndrome	متلازمه جيلن باري
Cardio Pulmonary Resuscitation CPR	الإنعاش القلبي ـ الرئوي
Alpha - 1 antitrypsin deficiency (glycoprotein)	نقص ألفا 1 ـ أنتي تريبسين
Bronchial asthma	الربو القصبي
Pulmonary edema	وذمة الرئة
Epiglotitis	التهاب لسان المزمار
Stridor	الصرير
Chronic Cough	السعال المزمن
Acute Bronchitis	مرض التهاب القصبات الحاد
Cystic Fibrosis - CF	التليف الكيسي الرئوي
Upper Respiratory Tract Infection	التهابات المجاري التنفسية العليا
Alveolar proteinosis (Surfactant)	داء الحويصلات الهوائية البروتيني
Diaphragm paralysis	شلل الحجاب الحاجز
Obstructive sleep apnea	متلازمة انقطاع التنفس الانسدادي أثناء النوم
Central sleep apnea	انقطاع التنفس المركزي أثناء النوم
Parasomnia	الأضطراب المصاحبة للنوم، خَطَلٌ نَوميّ الحديث والكلام والمشي أثناء النوم
Circadian rhythm disorder	اضطراب الساعة البيولوجية
hypnolepsy (= narcolepsy)	داء النوم الانتيابي (النوم المفرط بشكل مفاجيء)
Cataplexy	الجُمْدَة؛ نوبة مرضية فجائية
Sudden physical collapse though remaining conscious.	انهيار عصبي بسبب المشاعر القوية
Sudden muscles weakness, triggered by laugher or anger	

Investigations	
Diagnostic Service **Laboratory**	**المصطلح** **فحوصات المختبر (المعمل)**
CBC – Complete Blood Count (FBC – Full Blood Count)	تحليل تعداد الدم الكامل
TSH - Thyroid Stimulating Hormone	فحص الهرمون المنبه للغدة الدرقية
E.S.R (Erythrocyte Sedimentation Rate)	سرعة ترسب الكريات الحمراء أو سرعة ترسب الدم
CRP	اختبار البروتين المتفاعل
The C-reactive protein (CRP) test is a blood test that checks for inflammation in your body.	فحص الدم الذي يتحقق من وجود التهاب في جسمك.
Liver Function test	اختبارات وظائف الكبد
Creatinine	كرياتنين
Calcium	كالسيوم
Immonoglobin	الغلوبولين المناعي
IGE rast (for allergy)	فحص مستوى الأجسام المضادة من نوع IgE في مصل الدم
Serum ACE Angiotensin Converting Enzyme (ACE)	فحص انزيم الانجيوتنسين
Radiology	**أشعة**
Chest Xray	تصوير الصدر الإشعاعي
CT scan A computerized tomography (CT) scan	التصوير الطبقي المحوري للصدر (أشعة مقطعية)
CT pulmonary angiogram	التصوير الطبقي المحوري للشرايين الرئوية
Diaphragm screening	اختبار الحجاب الحاجز
Other tests	**فحوصات أخرى**
Spirometry , Breathing test	مقياس التنفس
Allergy Test (Skin Prick Test)	اختبار الحاسية (اختبار وخز الجلد)
Diagnostic Bronchoscopy	منظار القصبة الهوائية التشخيصي
Pulmonary Function Test (PFT) Studies	دراسات اختبار وظائف الرئة
Sleep Study Or Polysomnography (PSG)	دراسة النوم (مخطط النوم – اختبار النوم المتعدد)
DLCO – Diffusing Capacity Of The Lungs For Carbon Monoxide	سرعة انتشار غاز اول اكسيد الكربون خلال الغشاء التنفسي
Thoracentesis (pleural tap) is a procedure to remove excess fluid from the space between the lungs and the chest wall.	سحب السائل المتجمع في الحيز الجنبي
A pleural biopsy is a procedure to take a small piece of the pleura. This is done with a special biopsy	الخزعة الرئوية من الغشاء الجنبي

needle. Or it is done during surgery. The
biopsy is done to look for infection, cancer, or
another condition.

- **Skin Prick Test**

Skin Prick Test	
Allergens	المادة المُسبِّبَة للحساسية
Mite(2)	العثة (2)
D. Pteronyssinus (European House Dust Mite)	المُقْتَضِمَةُ المُنْتَسَّةُ (عث غبار المنزل الأوروبي)
D. Farinae (European House Dust Mite)	المُقْتَضِمَةُ الدَّقيقيَّةُ (عث غبار البيت الأوروبي)
Pollen (6)	حبوب اللقاح (6)
Bermuda Grass	عشب برمودا
Kentucky Bluegrass	عشب كنتاكي الأزرق
Orchard Grass	عشب المروج
Grass Mix	خليط من العشب
Common Ragweed	عشبة الخنازير
Date Palm	نخيل التمر (البلح)
Mold(3)	فطر العفن (3)
Alternaria Alternate (Tenius)	البديل البديل (تينوس)
Aspergillus Fumigates	دخان الرشاشيات
Cladosporium Mix (Fulvum, Herbar)	مزيج الكلادوسبوريوم (فولفوم ، أعشاب)
Epithelia (11)	ظهارة (1)
Cat Dander	وبر القط
Dog Dander	وبر الكلب
Rabbit Dander	وبر الأرنب
Cow Dander	وبر البقر
Horse Dander	وبر الحصان
Chicken Feather	ريش الدجاج
Duck Feather	ريشة البط
Budgerigar (Parakeet)	الببغاء (ببغاء)
Common Ant	النملة المشتركة
Fire Ant	نملة النار
German Cockroach	صرصور ألماني
Food (22)	المواد الغذائية (22)
Chicken Meat	لحم دجاج
Fish Mix	أنواع مختلفة من الأسماك
Shrimp	جمبري (الروبيان)
Cow Fresh Milk	حليب بقري طازج
Egg White	بياض البيضة
Egg Yolk	صفار البيض
Nuts	المكسرات

Almond	لوز
Hazelnut	بندق
Walnut	جوز
Cacao	الكاكاو
Sesame Seed	بذور السمسم
Fruits And Vegetable	فواكه وخضروات
Apple	التفاح
Banana	الموز
Orange	البرتقال
Peach	الخَوخ
Strawberry	الفراولة
Carrot	الجزر
Potato	البطاطس
Tomato	الطماطم
Barley Flour	دقيق الشعير
Wheat Flour	دقيق القمح
Other (1)	اخرى (1)
Latex	المطاط

- **Treatment**

Treatment	
Term	المصطلح
Medications	أدوية
Antibiotic medicine	المضادات الحيوية
Pain killer medicine	مسكن للألم
Antihistamine medicine	مضادات الهيستامين
Aerosol and humidity therapy– CPT, postural drainage and percussion (respiratory physiotherapy)	العلاج باستنشاق البخار والرطوبة – العلاج الطبيعي للصدر والنزح الوضعي والنقر (العلاج الطبيعي للجهاز التنفسي)
Asthma clinic including asthma education and rehabilitation	عيادة الربو وتشمل التوعية بمرض الربو وإعادة التأهيل
Bronchial hygiene therapy – CPT, postural drainage and percussion, Active Cycle of Breathing Therapy (ACBT) (respiratory physiotherapy)	العلاج بتنظيف الشعب الهوائية – العلاج الطبيعي للصدر والنزح الوضعي والنقر (العلاج الطبيعي للجهاز التنفسي)
Initiation and adjustment of CPAP machine	استخدام وضبط جهاز الضغط الإيجابي المستمر لمجرى الهواء
Therapeutic intervention bronchoscopy	منظار القصبة الهوائية العلاجي
Therapeutic sleep studies with CPAP/BIPAP therapy	دراسات النوم العلاجية باستخدام الضغط الإيجابي المستمر لمجرى الهواء / الضغط الإيجابي المستمر لمجرى الهواء من المستوى الثنائي
Treatment of respiratory disease	علاج أمراض الجهاز التنفسي
Inhaler	جهاز استنشاق
Nasal spray	بخاخ أنف
CPAP Machine	جهاز الضغط الإيجابي المستمر لمجرى الهواء
Nebulizer	جهاز البخار
Allergy tablets (antihistamine)	حبوب الحساسية
Antibiotic	مضادات حيوية
Sterioid (cortisone)	كورتيزون
Physiotherapy (to clear secretions and help to breath)	العلاج الطبيعي (للتخلص من الإفرازات والمساعدة على التنفس)
Oxygen intake,/ cylinder	أسطوانات اكسجين

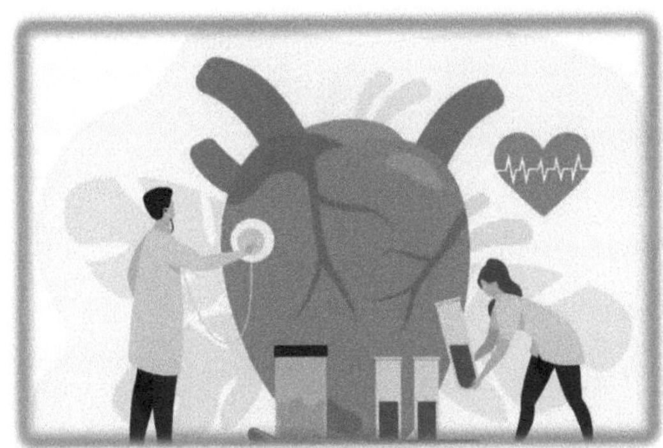

Chapter FIVE- Cardiology

Overview

This chapter introduces the reader to common medical terminology of Cardiology specialty that will include bilingual terminology for the following;

1. Anatomy
2. Common Symptoms
3. Diseases / Health Conditions
4. Further Diseases
5. Investigations
6. Assessment questions
7. Diseases and disorders
8. Treatment
9. Surgery / Procedures

We hope you enjoy reading this Chapter, and more chapters awaiting you

BLOOD CIRCULATION IN THE HEART

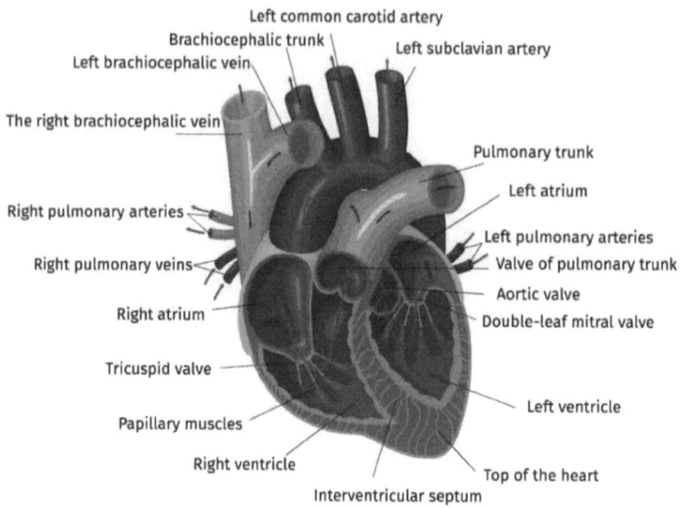

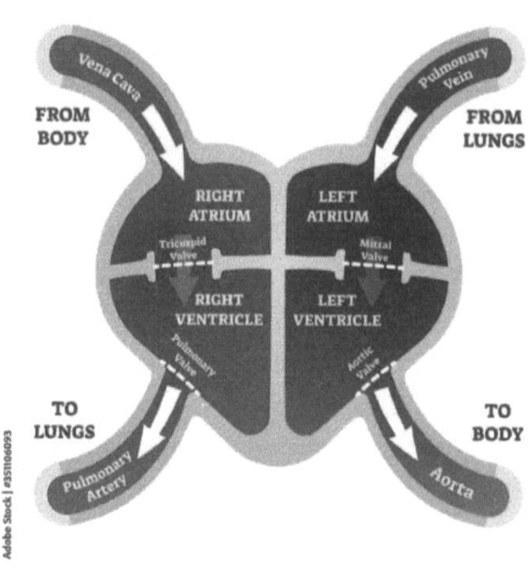

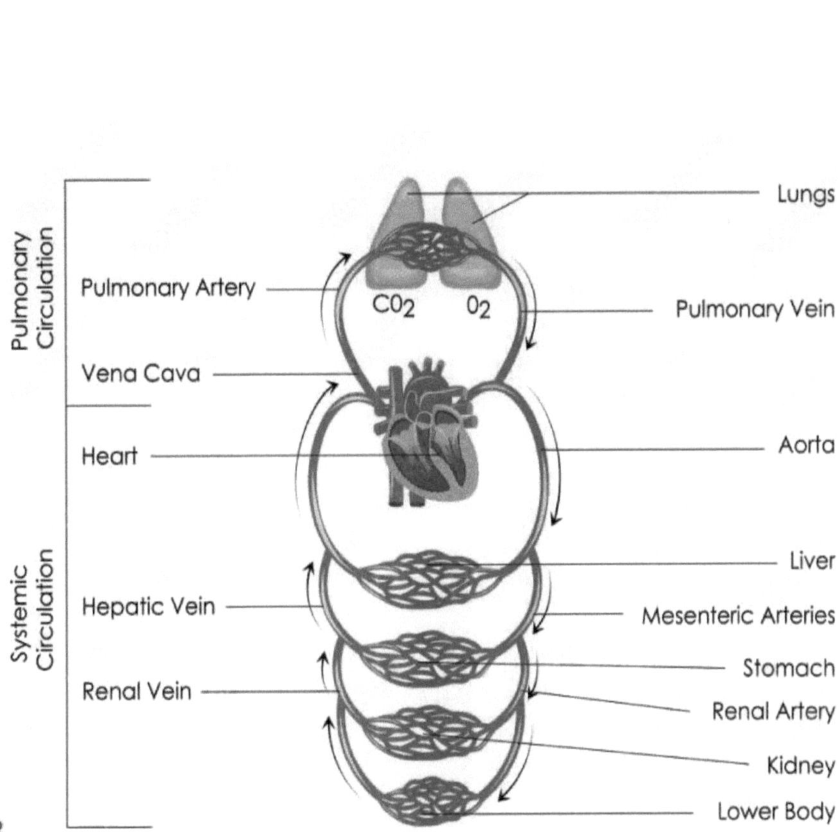

FLOW OF BLOOD

- The Common Symptoms

The Common Symptoms	
Term	**المصطلح**
Chest pain (angina).	ألم في الصدر (الذبحة الصدرية)
Chest pressure, heaviness or discomfort, sometimes described as a "belt around the chest" or a "weight on the chest."	ضغط على الصدر أو ثقله أو عدم ارتياح، ويوصف أحيانًا بأنه "حزام حول الصدر" أو "ثقل على الصدر."
Shortness of breath (dyspnea).	ضيق التنفس
Fatigue or exhaustion.	التعب أو الإرهاق.
Pain or cramps in your legs when you walk.	ألم أو تقلصات في ساقيك عند المشي.
Leg sores that are not healing.	تقرحات الساق التي لا تلتئم.
Cool or red skin on your legs.	برودة أو احمرار جلد الساق.
Numbness in your face or a limb. This may be on only one side of your body.	خدر في وجهك أو أحد أطرافك. قد يكون هذا في جانب واحد فقط من جسمك.
Difficulty with talking, seeing or walking	صعوبة في الكلام أو الرؤية أو المشي
Fainting (syncope).	الإغماء
Pain or numbness in your arms/legs.	ألم أو تنميل في ذراعيك / ساقيك.
Ripping or tearing chest or back pain.	آلام ممزقة وقاطعة في الصدر أو في الظهر.
Chest pain	ألم في الصدر
Pain in the neck, jaw, throat	ألم في الرقبة والفك والحلق
Pain in upper abdomen or back	ألم في أعلى البطن أو الظهر
Pain, numbness, weakness or coldness in the legs or arms if the blood vessels in those body areas are narrowed	ألم أو تنميل أو ضعف أو برودة في الساقين أو الذراعين في حال تضيق الأوعية الدموية في تلك المناطق من الجسم
Chest pain or discomfort	ألم أو عدم ارتياح في الصدر
Fainting (syncope)	الإغماء (فقدان الوعي)
near fainting	على وشك الإغماء
Fluttering in the chest/palpitation	رفرفة واضطراب في الصدر / خفقان
Lightheadedness	دوار (خفة في الرأس)
Racing heartbeat (tachycardia)	تسارع ضربات القلب
Slow heartbeat (bradycardia)	بطء ضربات القلب
Easily getting short of breath and tiring during exercise or activity	الشعور بضيق في التنفس والتعب بسهولة أثناء ممارسة الرياضة أو أي نشاط
Swelling of the hands, ankles or feet	تورم في اليدين أو الكاحلين أو القدمين
Pain, pressure, heaviness or discomfort in your chest or upper body.	ألم أو ضغط أو ثقل أو انزعاج في صدرك أو الجزء العلوي من جسمك.

Heartburn or indigestion.	حرقة في المعدة أو عسر الهضم.
Nausea or vomiting.	الغثيان (اللوعة) أو القيء.
Symptoms of heart pumping difficulties	مشاكل في عملية ضخ القلب
Exhaustion.	إنهاك.
Fatigue / tiredness	الإنهاك / التعب
Limitation of exercise capacity	محدودية القدرة على ممارسة الرياضة
Dizziness or sudden unexplained loss of consciousness.	الدوخة أو فقدان الوعي المفاجئ غير المبرر.
Inability to exercise.	عدم القدرة على ممارسة التمارين.
Sharp chest pain worse with deep inspiration.	ألم حاد في الصدر، يسوء مع التنفس العميق.
Chest pain with movement / twisting	ألم في الصدر مع الحركة / الالتواء
Chest pain worse when pressing on chest wall	ألم في الصدر أثناء الضغط على جدار الصدر

The Common Disease/health conditions	
Term	المصطلح
Abnormal heart rhythms, or arrhythmias	عدم انتظام ضربات القلب أو عدم انتظام نظم القلب
1. bradycardia or slow heart rate	1. بطء ضربات القلب
2. Tachycardia or fast heart rate	2. سرعة ضربات القلب
3. Atrial fibrillation (AF), irregular heart rhythm	3. الرجفان الأذيني (AF)، عدم انتظام ضربات القلب
4. Atrial flutter	4. الرفرفة الأذينية
5. Narrow complex supraventricular tachycardia	5. ضيق مُركب تسارع القلب فوق البطيني
6. Rapid ventricular tachycardia (VT)	6. تسارع القلب البطيني السريع (VT)
7. Ventricular fibrillation (VF)	7. الرجفان البطيني(VF)
8. Pulseless electrical activity (PEA)	8. النشاط الكهربائي غير النبضي (PEA)
9. Asystole	9. توقف الانقباض
Aortic disease and Marfan syndrome aneurysm (bulge) of the aorta	مرض الشريان الأورطي ومتلازمة مارفان تمدد الأوعية الدموية (انتفاخ) في الشريان الأورطي
Congenital heart disease (CHD)	أمراض القلب الخلقية (CHD)
▪ Atrial Septal Defect.	▪ عيب الحاجز الأذيني.
▪ Atrioventricular Septal Defect.	▪ عيب الحاجز الأذيني البطيني.
▪ Coarctation of the Aorta	▪ تضيق في الشريان الأورطي
▪ Double-outlet Right Ventricle	▪ البطين الأيمن مزدوج المخرج
▪ d-Transposition of the Great Arteries	▪ د- تبديل الشرايين الكبرى
▪ Ebstein Anomaly	▪ شذوذ إبشتاين
▪ Hypoplastic Left Heart Syndrome	▪ متلازمة القلب الأيسر الناقص التنسج
▪ Interrupted Aortic Arch	▪ قوس الأبهر المتقطع
Coronary artery disease (narrowing of the arteries); When plaque builds up and hardens the arteries. That hardening is also called atherosclerosis.	مرض الشريان التاجي (تضيق الشرايين). عندما تتراكم اللويحات وتصلب الشرايين. يسمى هذا التصلب أيضًا بتصلب الشرايين.
A. Angina	ذبحة الصدرية
▪ Stable angina – only on exercise	• الذبحة الصدرية المستقرة ـ فقط عند التمرين
▪ Unstable angina – symptoms at rest	• الذبحة الصدرية غير المستقرة ـ الأعراض أثناء الراحة
▪ Crescendo angina – rapidly increasing symptoms	• الذبحة الصدرية المتصاعدة ـ تتزايد الأعراض بسرعة
B. Heart attack; occurs when the flow of blood to the heart is severely reduced or blocked.	نوبة قلبية؛ يحدث عندما ينخفض أو يُسد تدفق الدم إلى القلب بشدة.
Heart failure; The heart does not pump as strongly as it should. This may cause your body to hold in salt and	سكتة قلبية (قصور القلب)؛ لا يضخ القلب بقوة كما ينبغي. سيؤدي ذلك إلى احتباس جسمك

water, which may cause leg swelling and shortness of breath.	للملح والماء ، مما يؤدي إلى انتفاخ الأرجل وضيق في التنفس.
Heart muscle disease (cardiomyopathy) (enlarged heart) (Thick Heart Muscle)	مرض عضلة القلب (اعتلال عضلة القلب) (تضخم القلب) (عضلة القلب السميكة)
Heart valves diseases;	أمرض صمامات القلب.
1. Aortic valve	الصمام الأبهر
■ Aortic stenosis (narrowed) Your aortic valve is narrowed. It slows blood flow from your heart to the rest of your body.	تضيق الأبهر. يضيق الصمام الأبهري. حيث يبطئ تدفق الدم من قلبك إلى باقي جسمك.
■ Aortic insufficiency (leaks) Aortic regurgitation (AR), also known as aortic insufficiency, is a form of valvular heart disease in which the integrity of the aortic valve is compromised and leads to inadequate closure of the valve leaflets. A normal aortic valve is comprised of three semilunar cusps that attach to the aortic wall.	قصور الأبهر (التسرب) قلس الأبهر (AR)، المعروف أيضًا باسم قصور الأبهر، هو شكل من أشكال أمراض القلب الصمامية التي تتعرض فيها سلامة الصمام الأبهري للخطر ويؤدي إلى إغلاق غير مناسب لوريقات الصمام. يتكون الصمام الأبهري الطبيعي من ثلاث شرفات هلالية متصلة بجدار الأبهر.
2. Mitral valve	الصمام التاجي (الميترالي)
■ Mitral valve insufficiency. Your mitral valve does not close tightly enough. This causes blood to leak backward, leading to fluid backup in the lungs.	قصور الصمام التاجي. لا يغلق الصمام التاجي بإحكام كافٍ. يؤدي هذا إلى تسرب الدم للخلف ، مما يؤدي إلى تراكم السوائل في الرئتين.
■ Mitral valve prolapse. The valve between your left upper and left lower chambers are not close correctly.	تدلي (انسدال) الصمام التاجي. الصمام الموجود بين الحجرة اليسرى العلوية واليسرى السفلية لا يغلق وجه صحيح.
3. Triscupid valve	صمام ثلاثي الشرف
■ Tricuspid regurgitation - Triscupid insufficiency (leaks) that occurs when the valve's flaps (cusps or leaflets) do not close properly. The tricuspid valve controls the flow of blood from your heart's right atrium (top chamber) to the right ventricle (bottom chamber).	قلس (قصور) صمام ثلاثي الشرف (التسرب) يحدث عندما لا تغلق سدائل الصمام (الشرفات أو الوريقات) بشكل صحيح. يتحكم الصمام ثلاثي الشرفات في تدفق الدم من الأذين الأيمن لقلبك (الغرفة العلوية) إلى البطين الأيمن (الغرفة السفلية).
■ Tricuspid stenosis (TS) (narrowed) is a very rare valvular abnormality occurring due to the narrowing of the tricuspid valve. It results in an elevated gradient between the right atrium and right ventricle, systemic congestion, and failure to augment right ventricle output	تضيق صمام ثلاثي الشرف هو شذوذ صمامي نادر جدًا يحدث نتيجة لتضييق الصمام ثلاثي الشرفات. يؤدي إلى ارتفاع التدرج بين الأذين الأيمن والبطين الأيمن، واحتقان هيكلي، وفشل في زيادة إنتاج البطين الأيمن
4. Pulmonary valve	الصمام الرئوي
■ Pulmonary stenosis (narrowed) that involves the narrowing of the pulmonary valve, which controls the flow of blood from the heart's right ventricle into the pulmonary artery to carry blood to the lungs.	تضيق الصمام الرئوي (تضيق) الذي ينطوي على تضيق الصمام الرئوي، الذي يتحكم في تدفق الدم من البطين الأيمن للقلب إلى الشريان الرئوي لنقل الدم إلى الرئتين.
■ Pulmonary valve regurgitation occurs when the pulmonary valve doesn't completely close and allows some blood to leak back into the heart. This condition is also known	ارتجاع الصمام الرئوي يحدث عندما لا ينغلق الصمام الرئوي بشكل كامل ويسمح لبعض الدم بالتسرب مرة أخرى إلى القلب. تُعرف هذه الحالة أيضًا باسم القلس الرئوي والقصور الرئوي والقصور الرئوي.

as pulmonic regurgitation, pulmonic insufficiency and pulmonary insufficiency.	
Rheumatic heart disease	مرض روماتيزم القلب
An inflammatory disease that usually was in childhood following a sore throat, that can damage your heart valves.	أحد الأمراض الالتهابية الأكثر شيوعًا عند الأطفال ، ويؤدي إلى تلف صمامات القلب.
Stroke	سكتة دماغية
Blockage of blood flow to your brain, which can cause visual disturbance, speech abnormality or weakness / numbness on one side	عامل يبطئ أو يمنع تدفق الدم إلى دماغك والتي يمكن أن تسبب اضطرابًا في الرؤية أو خللًا في الكلام أو ضعفًا / تنميلًا في جانب واحد
Peripheral vascular disease	أمراض الأوعية الدموية الطرفية
Reduced circulation of blood (usually affecting legs and feet)	انخفاض الدورة الدموية (عادة يؤثر على القدم والأرجل)
Deep vein thrombosis and pulmonary embolism(DVT)	تجلط الأوردة العميقة (الجلطة الرئوية)

- Further Diseases / Health Conditions

Term	المصطلح
Further Disease/health conditions	
▪ Adult Congenital Heart Disease	▪ أمراض القلب الخلقية لدى البالغين
▪ Heart Failure/Cardiomyopathy	▪ فشل القلب / اعتلال عضلة القلب
▪ Alcohol Septal Ablation	▪ استئصال الحاجز الكحولي
▪ Amyloid Heart Disease	▪ مرض القلب النشواني
▪ Aneurysm: Abdominal	▪ تمدد الأوعية الدموية: البطن
▪ Aneurysm: Aortic	▪ تمدد الأوعية الدموية: الأبهر
▪ Aneurysm: Thoracic	▪ تمدد الأوعية الدموية: الصدري
▪ Aneurysm: Peripheral	▪ تمدد الأوعية الدموية: المحيطي
▪ Aneurysm Repair	▪ إصلاح تمدد الأوعية الدموية
▪ Aortic Disease	▪ مرض الشريان الأورطي
▪ Atherosclerosis	▪ تصلب الشرايين
▪ Atrial Fibrillation	▪ رجفان أذيني
▪ Cardiac Ablation	▪ عملية كي التسارعات القلبية
▪ Cardiac Amyloidosis	▪ داء النشواني القلبي
▪ Cardiac Arrhythmia	▪ عدم انتظام ضربات القلب
▪ Cardiac Catheterization	▪ قسطرة القلب
▪ Tumors of the Heart	▪ أورام القلب
▪ Cardiovascular Genetic Diseases	▪ الأمراض الوراثية القلبية الوعائية
▪ Carotid Angioplasty and Stenting	▪ رأب الوعاء السباتي باستخدام الدعامات
▪ Carotid Disease	▪ مرض الشريان السباتي
▪ Carotid Endarterectomy	▪ استئصال باطنة الشريان السباتي
▪ Cerebrovascular Disease	▪ مرض الأوعية الدموية الدماغية
▪ Coronary Angioplasty and Stenting	▪ رأب الأوعية التاجية باستخدام الدعامات
▪ Coronary Artery Bypass Grafting (CABG)	▪ تطعيم مجازة الشريان التاجي (CABG)
▪ Coronary Heart Disease	▪ مرض القلب التاجي
▪ Deep Vein Thrombosis and Pulmonary Embolism	▪ تجلط الأوردة العميقة والتجلط الرئوي
▪ Dialysis Access or fistula	▪ مدخل إلى غسيل الكلى
▪ Embolectomy	▪ استئصال الصمة
▪ Endocarditis	▪ التهاب داخلي بالقلب
▪ Endovascular Repair	▪ إصلاح الأوعية الدموية
▪ Extracorporeal Membrane Oxygenation (ECMO)	▪ أكسجة الغشاء خارج الجسم (ECMO)
▪ Heart Rhythm Disorders	▪ اضطرابات نظم القلب
▪ Heart Valve Disease	▪ مرض صمام القلب
▪ Hyperlipidemia (High Blood Cholesterol) and Obesity	▪ فرط شحميات الدم (ارتفاع نسبة الكوليسترول في الدم) والسمنة
▪ Hypertension (High Blood Pressure)	▪ ارتفاع ضغط الدم (ارتفاع ضغط الدم)
▪ Implantable Cardiac Defibrillator (ICD)	▪ مزيل الرجفان القلبي القابل للزرع (ICD)
▪ Pacemaker implantation	▪ زرع جهاز تنظيم ضربات القلب
▪ Pericardial Disease	▪ مرض التامور

- Peripheral Artery Disease (PAD)	مرض الشريان المحيطي (PAD) -
- Peripheral Bypass Surgery	جراحة المجازة الطرفية -
- Pregnancy and Heart Disease	الحمل وأمراض القلب -
- Prevention of Heart and Vascular Disease	الوقاية من أمراض القلب والأوعية الدموية -
- Pulmonary Hypertension	ارتفاع ضغط الشريان الرئوي -
- Pulmonary Embolism	التجلط الرئوي -
- Pulmonary Vascular Disease	أمراض الأوعية الدموية الرئوية -
- Renal Artery Stenosis	تضيق الشريان الكلوي -
- Septal Myectomy	استئصال عضلة الحاجز -
- Stent Graft	زرع دعامات -
- Structural Heart Disease	أمراض القلب الهيكلية -
- Thoracic Outlet Syndrome	متلازمة مخرج الصدر -
- Thromboendarterectomy	استئصال الخثرة -
- Thrombolytic Therapy	علاج التخثر -
- Transcatheter Aortic Valve Replacement (TAVR)	استبدال الصمام الأبهري عبر القسطرة (TAVR) -
- Transvenous pacemaker lead Extraction	استخراج أسلاك جهاز تنظيم ضربات القلب عن طريق الوريد -
- Varicose Vein Treatment	علاج الدوالي -
- Venous and Lymphatic Disorders	الاضطرابات الوريدية واللمفاوية -
- Ventricular Assist Device (VAD)	أجهزة المساعدة البطينية (VADs) -
- Ventricular Tachycardia	تسارع القلب البطيني -
- Aortic stenosis /regurgitation or insufficiency	تضيق الأبهر(الأورطى) / قلس أو قصور -
- Mitral stenosis /regurgitation	تضيق / قلس المترالي /ارتجاع الصمام المترالي -
- Pulmonary stenosis/regurgitation	تضيق / ارتجاع رئوي -
- Tricuspid stenosis /regurgitation	تضيق / ارتجاع صمام ثلاثي الشرفات -

- **Investigations**

Investigations	
Diagnostic Service Laboratory	المصطلح فحوصات المختبر (المعمل)
Blood work; measures substances that indicate cardiovascular health, such as cholesterol, blood sugar levels and specific proteins. A provider can use a blood test to check for blood clotting issues as well.	فحوصات الدم يقيس المواد التي تشير إلى صحة القلب والأوعية الدموية ، مثل الكوليسترول ومستويات السكر في الدم وبروتينات معينة. يمكن للمزود استخدام فحص الدم للتحقق من مشاكل تخثر الدم أيضًا.
Ankle brachial index (ABI); compares the blood pressure in your ankles and arms to diagnose peripheral artery disease.	مؤشر الكاحل العضدي (ABI) يقارن ضغط الدم في الكاحلين والذراعين لتشخيص مرض الشريان المحيطي.
Non-Invasive Lab Services	الخدمات غير تداخلية
Electrocardiogram (EKG / ECG) records your heart's electrical activity.	مخطط كهربية القلب.(ECG) يسجل النشاط الكهربائي لقلبك.
Ambulatory monitoring; uses wearable devices that track your heart rhythm and rates. 24 Ambulatory Holter and blood pressure monitoring	مراقبة متنقلة لتخطيط كهربية القلب يستخدم أجهزة يمكن ارتداؤها لتعقب إيقاع قلبك ومعدلاته. جهاز هولتر لرصد تخطيط كهربية القلب خلال 24 ساعة, ومراقبة ضغط الدم
Echocardiogram (ECHO) ; uses sound waves to create an image of your heartbeat and blood flow.	مخطط صدى القلب (ECHO) ؛ يستخدم الموجات الصوتية لإنشاء صورة لضربات قلبك وتدفق الدم.
Ultrasound; uses sound waves to check blood flow in your legs or neck.	الموجات فوق الصوتية. يستخدم الموجات الصوتية للتحقق من تدفق الدم في ساقيك أو رقبتك.
Exercise Tolerance Test (Treadmill test)	اختبار تحمل الإجهاد (اختبار جهاز المشي)
Stress Echocardiography	تصوير القلب الصدوي الإجهادي
Stress tests; analyze how physical activity affects your heart in a controlled setting, using exercise or medications, to determine how your heart responds. This type of test can involve EKGs and/or imaging tests.	اختبارات الإجهاد: تحليل كيفية تأثير النشاط البدني على قلبك في بيئة خاضعة للتعقب ، باستخدام التمارين أو الأدوية ، لتحديد كيفية استجابة قلبك. يمكن أن يشمل هذا النوع من الاختبارات تخطيط كهربية القلب و / أو اختبارات التصوير.
Invasive Cath-Lab services	الخدمات التداخلية
Coronary and peripheral angiography	تصوير الأوعية التاجية والمحيطية
Coronary and peripheral angioplasty	رأب الأوعية التاجية والمحيطية
Right heart catheterization	اختبار ضخ القلب للدم
Permanent pacemaker implantation	زرع جهاز منظم ضربات القلب الدائم
Permanent pacemaker interrogation	فحص جهاز منظم ضربات القلب الدائم

Biventricular Pacemaker for heart failure (cardiac resynchronization therapy)	منظم ضربات القلب ثنائي البطينين لعلاج فشل القلب (علاج إعادة التزامن القلبي)
Implantable cardioverter defibrillator (ICD) implantation	زرع جهاز مقوم نظم القلب ومزيل الرجفان (ICD)
Implantable cardioverter defibrillator (ICD) interrogation	التحقق من عمل مقوم نظم القلب ومزيل الرجفان (ICD) المزروع
Cardiac computerized tomography (CT); uses X-rays and computer processing to create 3D images of your heart and blood vessels.	التصوير المقطعي المحوسب للقلب (CT) ؛ يستخدم الأشعة السينية ومعالجة الكمبيوتر لإنشاء صور ثلاثية الأبعاد للقلب والأوعية الدموية.
Cardiac magnetic resonance imaging (MRI); uses magnetic fields and radio waves to create highly detailed images of your heart.	التصوير بالرنين المغناطيسي للقلب (MRI) ؛ يستخدم موجات مغناطيسية وموجات الراديو لإنشاء صور مفصلة للغاية لقلبك.
Stress cardiac MRI; uses a medication to increase blood flow and look for coronary artery narrowings	فحص القلبي بالرنين المغناطيسي. يستخدم دواء لزيادة تدفق الدم والبحث عن تضيق الشريان التاجي
MR angiogram or CT angiogram; uses an MRI or CT, respectively, to see blood vessels in your legs, head and neck.	تصوير الأوعية بالرنين المغناطيسي أو التصوير الوعائي المقطعي المحوسب ؛ يستخدم التصوير بالرنين المغناطيسي أو التصوير المقطعي المحوسب ، على التوالي ، لرؤية الأوعية الدموية في ساقيك ورأسك ورقبتك.
Cardiac catheterization; uses a catheter (thin, hollow tube) to measure pressure and blood flow in your heart. And look at the coronary arteries	قسطرة القلب؛ يستخدم قسطرة (أنبوب رفيع مجوف) لقياس الضغط وتدفق الدم في قلبك. وفحص الشرايين التاجية
Coronary artery intervention; you may need a procedure to implant a stent to open up a blocked or narrowed coronary artery.	إدخال الشريان التاجي : قد تحتاج إلى إجراء لزرع دعامة لفتح الشريان التاجي المسدود أو الضيق.

- **Assessment questions**

A. How far can you walk?
- <100m
- 100m
- >100m

B. Do you get short of breath/breathless?
- No, no limitation of physical activity
- Yes, mild limitation on exercise. Comfortable at rest
- Yes, marked limitation on exercise. Comfortable at rest
- Yes, unable to do any exercise due to breathlessness or breathless at rest.

C. Do you get chest discomfort/tightness/pain?
- No
- On strenuous exercise
- With mild/minimal exercise
- At rest

D. Does the chest discomfort subside when you stop exercise? When you use GTN (glyceryl trinitrate (GTN) tablets and spray under your tongue.

E. Do you have.......
- Diabetes Type (on insulin), Type 2
- High blood pressure
- Family history of heart attack/stent/coronary artery disease/stroke/sudden death
- High cholesterol
- Current or previous history of smoking
- Previous history of heart attack or other cardiac condition.

- **Treatment**

Treatment	
Term	**المصطلح**
Lifestyle changes:	**تغيير نمط الحياة:**
Change your diet – eat healthy	غيّر نظامك الغذائي ـ تناول طعامًا صحيًا
Lose weight	فقدان الوزن
Increase aerobic exercise	زيادة التمارين الهوائية الإيروبيك)
Quit smoking/tobacco products	الإقلاع عن التدخين / منتجات التبغ
Medications:	**الأدوية:**
Your healthcare provider may prescribe medications to help manage cardiovascular disease. Medication type will depend on what kind of cardiovascular disease you have.	قد يصف مقدم الرعاية الصحية الخاص بك الأدوية للمساعدة في إدارة أمراض القلب والأوعية الدموية. يعتمد نوع الدواء على نوع مرض القلب والأوعية الدموية الذي تعاني منه.
Procedures or surgeries:	**الإجراءات أو العمليات الجراحية:**
If medications are not enough, your healthcare provider may use certain procedures or surgeries to treat your cardiovascular disease. Examples include stents in your heart or leg arteries, minimally invasive heart surgery, open-heart surgery, ablations or cardioversion.	إذا لم تكن الأدوية كافية ، فقد يستخدم مقدم الرعاية الصحية الخاص بك بعض الإجراءات أو العمليات الجراحية لعلاج أمراض القلب والأوعية الدموية. تشمل الأمثلة الدعامات في شرايين القلب أو الساق ، أو جراحة القلب طفيفة التوغل ، أو جراحة القلب المفتوح ، أو الاجتثاث ، أو تقويم نظم القلب.
Cardiac rehabilitation:	إعادة تأهيل القلب:
You may need a monitored exercise program to help your heart get stronger.	قد تحتاج إلى برنامج تمرين خاضع للمراقبة لمساعدة قلبك على أن يصبح أقوى.
Active surveillance:	المراقبة النشطة:
You may need careful monitoring over time without medications or procedures/surgeries.	قد تحتاج إلى مراقبة دقيقة بمرور الوقت بدون أدوية أو إجراءات / جراحات.
Aortic Root Repair/Replacement	إصلاح /استبدال جذر الأبهر
Aortic Valve Repair/Replacement	إصلاح /استبدال الصمام الأبهري
Cardiac CT	التصوير المقطعي المحوسب للقلب
Cardiac Magnetic Resonance Imaging	التصوير بالرنين المغناطيسي للقلب
Cardiac Resynchronization Therapy	علاج إعادة تزامن القلب
Cardiac Ultrasound (Echocardiography)	الموجات فوق الصوتية للقلب (تخطيط صدى القلب)
Heart Transplant	زرع قلب
Minimally Invasive Cardiac Surgery	جراحة القلب طفيفة التوغل
Mitral Valve Repair and Replacement	إصلاح واستبدال الصمام التاجي
pacemaker implantation	زرع أجهزة تنظيم ضربات القلب
Complex pacemaker implant for heart failure	زرع منظم ضربات القلب المعقد لفشل القلب
ICD implant (Implantable cardioverter-defibrillator)	زرع ICD (مقوم نظم القلب ومزيل الرجفان القابل للزراعة)

Coronary artery intervention/stenting	تدخل / تركيب دعامة للشريان التاجي
Standard Exercise Tolerance Test	اختبار تحمل التمرين القياسي
Vascular Imaging	تصوير الأوعية الدموية

An ICD is a battery-powered device placed under the skin that keeps track of your heart rate. Thin wires connect the ICD to the heart. If an abnormal heart rhythm is detected the device will try to correct the heart rhythm It may need to deliver an electric shock to restore a normal heartbeat if the heart is beating chaotically and much too fast.

Surgery / Procedures	
Term	المصطلح
Implantable Cardioverter Defibrillator (ICD) An ICD is a battery-powered device placed under the skin that keeps track of your heart rate. Thin wires connect the ICD to the heart. If an abnormal heart rhythm is detected the device will try to correct the heart rhythm It may need to deliver an electric shock to restore a normal heartbeat if the heart is beating chaotically and much too fast. ICDs have been very useful in preventing sudden death in patients with known, sustained ventricular tachycardia or fibrillation. Studies have shown that they may have a role in preventing cardiac arrest in high-risk patients who have not had, but are at risk for, life-threatening ventricular arrhythmias.	زراعة جهاز مزيل رجفان القلب جهاز مقوم نظم القلب ومزيل الرجفان القابل للزراعة هو جهاز يعمل بالبطارية يوضع تحت الجلد ويتتبع معدل ضربات قلبك. تربط الأسلاك الرفيعة جهاز مقوم نظم القلب ومزيل الرجفان القابل للزراعة بالقلب. إذا تم اكتشاف إيقاع غير طبيعي في القلب ، فسيحاول الجهاز تصحيح إيقاع القلب ، وقد يحتاج إلى توصيل صدمة كهربائية لاستعادة نبضات القلب الطبيعية إذا كان القلب ينبض بشكل فوضوي وبسرعة كبيرة. أصبحت أجهزة تنظيم ضربات القلب ذات أهمية بالغة في الوقاية من حالات الموت المفاجئ لدى المرضى الذين يعانون من عدم انتظام دقات القلب أو الرجفان البطيني، كما وقد أظهرت الدراسات أنه قد يكون لها دور في الوقاية من السكتة القلبية لدى المرضى الذين لم يصابوا من قبل بعدم انتظام دقات القلب البطيني المهددة للحياة والمعرضين في نفس الوقت لخطر الإصابة به.
Pacemaker A pacemaker is a small device that helps the heart beat more regularly. It does this with a small electric stimulation. The doctor puts the pacemaker under the skin on the chest, just under the collarbone. It is connected to the heart with small wires. You may need a pacemaker to keep the heart beating properly.	جهاز تنظيم ضربات القلب جهاز تنظيم ضربات القلب هو جهاز صغير يساعد على تنظيم ضربات القلب. يقوم الجهاز بهذه الوظيفة من خلال إرسال محفزات كهربائية. يزرع الطبيب جهاز تنظيم ضربات القلب تحت الجلد في منطقة الصدر تحت الترقوة. يتم توصيل الجهاز بأسلاك توصيل كهربائية رفيعة. قد يحتاج المريض إلى جهاز تنظيم ضربات القلب للحفاظ على ضربات القلب بشكل إيقاعي منتظم.
Cardiac Resynchronization Therapy (CRT) Patients with heart failure may have an abnormal or dyssynchronous pattern of heart muscle contraction. In theses patient's, Cardiac Resynchronization Therapy (CRT) Patients CRT, or biventricular pacing, is used to help improve the heart's pumping function and the symptoms associated with heart failure. The procedure involves implanting a device, usually just below the collarbone. Three wires	جهاز علاج اختلال التزامن القلبي المرضى الذين يعانون من قصور القلب قد يكون لديهم نمط غير طبيعي أو غير متزامن لتقلص عضلة القلب. في حالة المريض ، يتم استخدام CRT (علاج إعادة التزامن القلبي CRT) ، أو تنظيم البطينين ، للمساعدة في تحسين وظيفة ضخ القلب والأعراض المرتبطة بفشل القلب. يتضمن الإجراء زرع جهاز، وعادة ما يكون أسفل عظم الترقوة. ثلاثة أسلاك (أسلاك) متصلة بالجهاز تراقب معدل ضربات القلب لتحسين وظائف القلب.

(leads) connected to the device monitor the heart rate to improve heart function.

<table>
<tr><td colspan="2">

Congenital Heart Disease and Heart Surgery

</td></tr>
</table>

Atrial Septal Defect (ASD)

This is a hole in the wall (septum) that separates the two upper chambers of the heart. This defect allows oxygen-rich blood to leak from the left side of the heart into the right side. A small hole may close on its own, but a larger one usually requires device closure or surgery.

عيب الحاجز الأذيني (ASD)

هذا هو ثقب في الجدار (الحاجز) الذي يفصل بين الحجرتين العلويتين من القلب. يسمح هذا العيب للدم الغني بالأكسجين بالتسرب من الجانب الأيسر للقلب إلى الجانب الأيمن. قد يُغلق الثقب الصغير من تلقاء نفسه ، لكن الثقب الأكبر يتطلب عادةً إغلاق الجهاز أو الجراحة.

Ventricular Septal Defect (VSD)

This defect involves a hole in the wall (septum) separating the two lower chambers of the heart. Oxygen-rich blood gets pumped back to the lungs instead of out to the body, causing the heart to pump harder. A small hole may close on its own, but a larger one usually requires device closure or surgery.

عيب الحاجز البطيني (VSD)

يتضمن هذا العيب وجود ثقب في الجدار (الحاجز) الذي يفصل بين غرفتي القلب السفليتين. ثم يُضخ الدم الغني بالأكسجين مرة أخرى إلى الرئتين بدلاً من خروجه إلى الجسم ، مما يؤدي إلى ضخ القلب بقوة أكبر. قد يُغلق الثقب الصغير من تلقاء نفسه ، لكن الثقب الأكبر يتطلب عادةً إغلاق الجهاز أو الجراحة.

Transposition Of The Great Arteries (TGA)

In this heart defect, which is present at birth, the two main arteries leading out of the heart, the pulmonary artery and the aorta, are switched in position or transposed. There are different types, some of which need surgery as an infant and some are only picked up later in life.

تبديل الشرايين الكبرى (TGA)

في هذا العيب القلبي ، الموجود عند الولادة ، يتم تبديل الشريانين الرئيسيين الخارجين من القلب ، الشريان الرئوي والشريان الأورطي ، في موضعهما أو يتم تبديل موضعهما. هناك أنواع مختلفة ، بعضها يحتاج إلى عملية جراحية للرضيع والبعض الآخر لا يتم التعرف عليه إلا في وقت لاحق من الحياة.

Atrioventricular (AV) Canal Defect

This defect is a large hole in the center of the heart. It is located where the wall (septum) between the upper chambers (atria) joins the wall between the lower chambers (ventricles). This septal defect involves both upper and lower chambers. Also, the tricuspid and mitral valves that normally separate the heart's upper and lower chambers may not be formed as individual valves. Instead, a single large valve forms that crosses the defect in the wall between the two sides of the heart. This often needs surgical correction in childhood.

عيب في القناة الأذينية البطينية

هو ثقب كبير في وسط القلب. يقع حيث يربط الجدار (الحاجز) بين الحجرتين العلويتين (الأذينين) بالجدار بين الغرف السفلية (البطينين). يشمل هذا العيب الحاجز كلا من الحجرات العلوية والسفلية. أيضًا ، لا يتم تكوين الصمامات ثلاثية الشرفات والصمامات التاجية التي تفصل عادةً بين حجرات القلب العلوية والسفلية كصمامات فردية. بدلاً من ذلك ، يتشكل صمام كبير واحد يعبر العيب في الجدار بين جانبي القلب. هذا غالبًا ما يحتاج إلى تصحيح جراحي في مرحلة الطفولة.

Coarctation of the aorta

In this condition the aorta (the main artery that carries blood from the heart to the body) is narrowed or constricted.

In most patients, the cause is not known. Some people can have other heart defects along with coarctation (such as a biscupid aortic valve).

Coarctation obstructs blood flow from the heart to the lower part of the body. Blood pressure increases above the constriction.

Tetralogy of Fallot

This is a combination of four heart defects that are present at birth (congenital).

These defects, which affect the structure of the heart, cause oxygen-poor blood to flow out of the heart and to the rest of the body. Infants and children with tetralogy of Fallot might have blue-tinged skin because their blood does not carry enough oxygen.

Tetralogy of Fallot is often diagnosed during infancy or soon after. However, tetralogy of Fallot might not be detected until later in life in some adults, depending on the severity of the defects and symptoms. Patients who have had surgery as children will need ongoing surveillance as adults.

تضيق في الشريان الأورطي

في هذه الحالة ، يضيق الشريان الأورطي (الشريان الرئيسي الذي ينقل الدم من القلب إلى الجسم) أو يتقلص.

في معظم المرضى ، السبب غير معروف. يمكن أن يعاني بعض الأشخاص من عيوب قلبية أخرى مع تضيق الأبهر (مثل الصمام الأبهري ثنائي الشرف).

يعيق التضيق تدفق الدم من القلب إلى الجزء السفلي من الجسم. يزيد ضغط الدم فوق الانقباض.

رباعية فالو

ناتج عن مجموعة من أربعة عيوب في القلب كانت موجودة عند الولادة (خلقي)

تؤدي هذه العيوب ، التي تؤثر على بنية القلب ، إلى تدفق الدم المحتوي على الأكسجين من القلب وإلى باقي الجسم. قد يكون للرضع والأطفال المصابين برباعية فالو جلد مزرق اللون لأن دمهم لا يحمل كمية كافية من الأكسجين.

غالبًا ما يتم تشخيص رباعية فالو خلال فترة الرضاعة أو بعدها بفترة وجيزة. ومع ذلك ، قد لا يتم اكتشاف رباعية فالو إلا في وقت لاحق من الحياة لدى بعض البالغين ، اعتمادًا على شدة العيوب والأعراض.

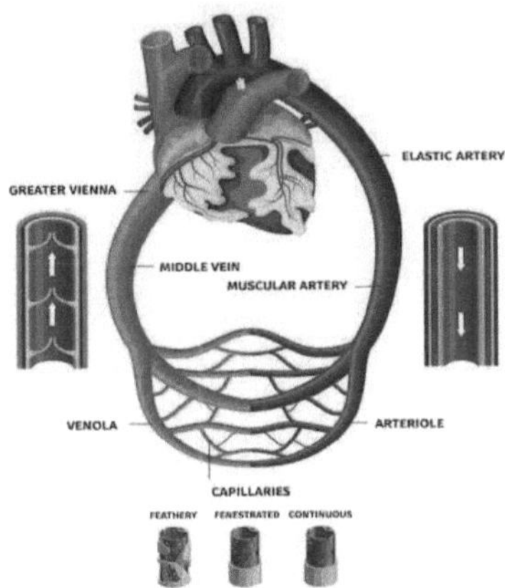

Chapter SIX- Vascular

Overview

This chapter introduces the reader to common medical terminology of Vascular specialty that will include bilingual terminology for the following;

1. Anatomy
2. Common Symptoms
3. Diseases / Health Conditions
4. Further Diseases
5. Investigations
6. Treatment
7. Surgery / Procedures
8. Complications

We hope you enjoy reading this Chapter, and more chapters awaiting you

Arteries and Veins of the Leg

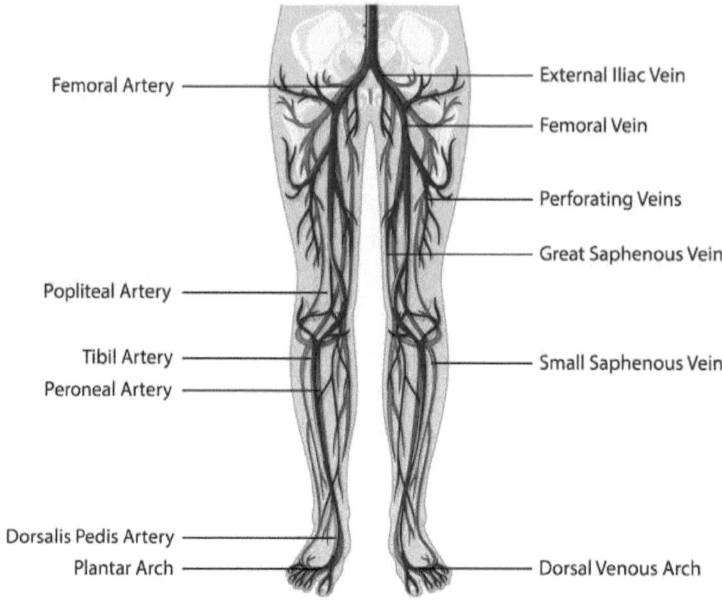

Circulatory System

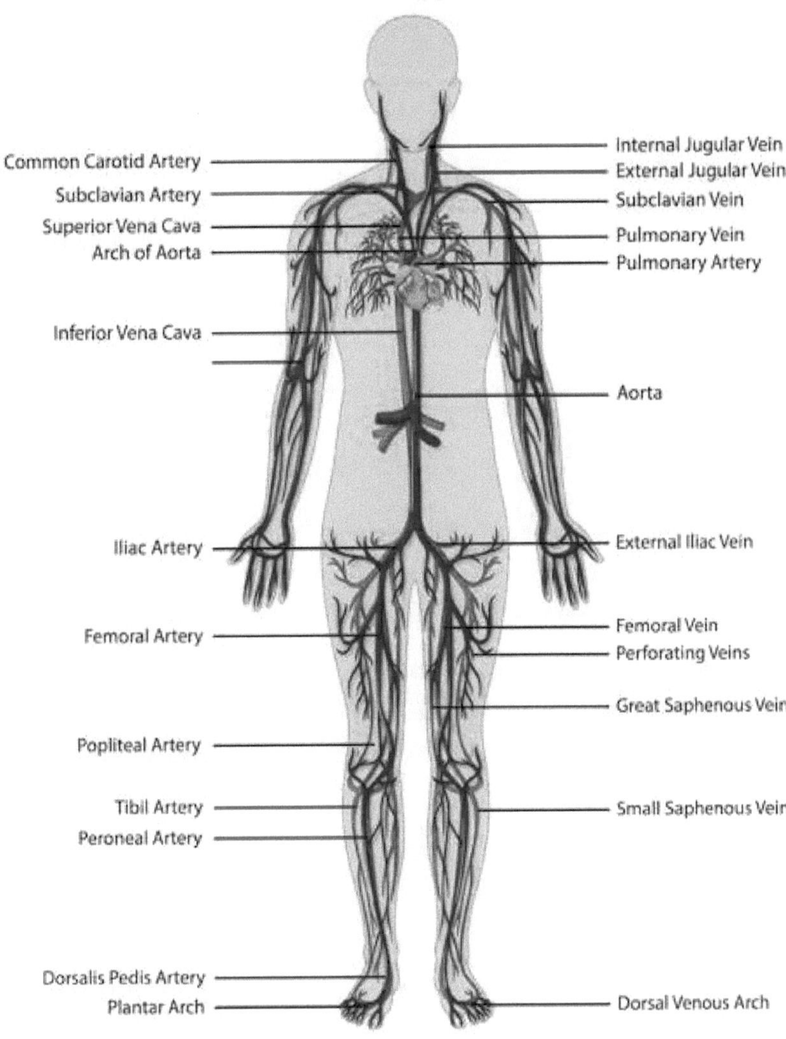

Your vascular system – the highways of the body – is composed of three types of blood vessels.

Arteries	Veins	Capillaries
Arteries carry oxygen-rich blood from the heart, nourishing every part of the body. The one exception is the pulmonary artery, which carries oxygen-poor blood from your heart to your lungs, where it exchanges carbon dioxide for oxygen.	Veins carry the blood back to the heart where it is replenished with oxygen. The newly oxygen-rich blood gets pumped back into the heart via the pulmonary vein.	Capillaries connect the arteries to the veins. Vascular disease commonly occurs at sites of unstable blood flow. For example, when the blood flow in the arteries changes direction suddenly.

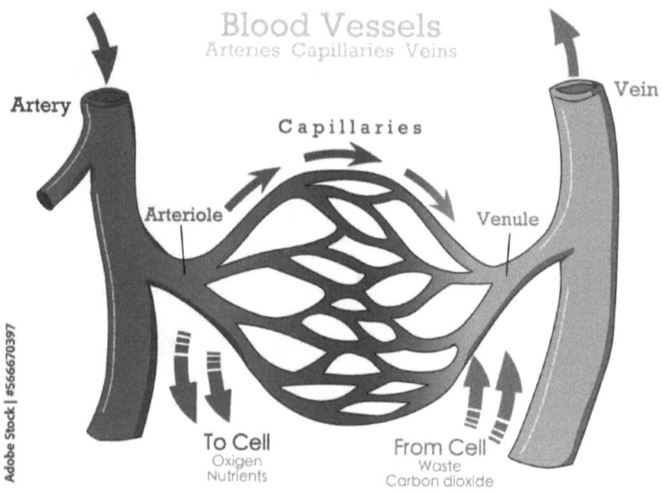

- **The Common Symptoms**

The Common Symptoms	
Term	**المصطلح**
Pain	ألم
Abnormal color changes in the fingertips	تغيرات غير طبيعية في لون أطراف الأصابع
Ulcers or wounds that do not heal	القرحات أو الجروح التي لا تلتئم
Hand pain when in cold temperatures or locations	ألم اليد في حالات انخفاض درجات الحرارة أو بالأماكن الباردة
Numbness or tingling in the fingertips	خدر أو وخز في أطراف الأصابع
Swelling	تورم
Cool or cold fingers and/or hands	برودة الأصابع و/ أو اليدين
Angina (chest pain)	الذبحة الصدرية (ألم في الصدر)
Heaviness, tightness, pressure, burning, or pain in the chest behind the breastbone	ثقل أو ضيق أو ضغط أو حرقان أو ألم في الصدر خلف عظم الصدر
Pain spreading to the arms, shoulders, jaw, neck, or back	ينتشر الألم إلى الذراعين أو الكتفين أو الفك أو الرقبة أو الظهر
Weakness and severe tiredness (fatigue) especially during periods of activity	الضعف والتعب الشديد (إنهاك) خاصة أثناء فترات النشاط
Nausea	غثيان
Sweating	التعرق
Pale or bluish skin	جلد شاحب أو مزرق
Lack of leg hair or toenail growth	قلة شعر الساق أو نمو أظافر القدم
Sores on toes, feet, or legs that heal slowly or not at all	تقرحات في أصابع القدم أو القدمين أو الساقين والتي تلتئم ببطء أو لا تلتئم على الإطلاق
Decreased skin temperature, or thin, brittle, shiny skin on the legs and feet	انخفاض درجة حرارة الجلد، أو ترقق ولمعان وهشاشة الجلد في منطقة الساقين والقدمين
Weak pulses in the legs and the feet	نبضات ضعيفة في الساقين والقدمين
Impotence	ضعف جنسي
Wounds that won't heal over pressure points, such as heels or ankles	الجروح التي لا تلتئم عند نقاط الضغط ، مثل الكعب أو الكاحلين
Numbness, weakness, or heaviness in muscles	خدر أو ضعف أو ثقل في العضلات
Burning or aching pain at rest, commonly in the toes and at night while lying flat	ألم حارق أو وجع أثناء الراحة ، عادةً في أصابع القدم وفي الليل أثناء الاستلقاء
Restricted mobility	تقيد ومحدودية الحركة
Thickened, opaque toenails	أظافر القدم السميكة وغير الشفافة
Varicose veins	توسع الأوردة (دوالي الأوردة)
Pain in the jaw, neck, or upper back	ألم في الفك أو الرقبة أو أعلى الظهر

Pain in the chest or back	ألم في الصدر أو الظهر
Wheezing, coughing, or shortness of breath	التنفس بصفير، أزيز أو سعال أو ضيق في التنفس
Hoarseness as a result of pressure on the vocal cords	بحة في الصوت نتيجة الضغط على الحبال الصوتية
skin infections	عدوى الجلد
skin ulcers	تقرحات الجلد
severe pain in the affected limb	ألم شديد في الطرف المصاب
paleness or coldness of the affected limb	شحوب أو برودة الطرف المصاب
numbness or weakness of the affected limb	خدر أو ضعف في الطرف المصاب
intense stomach pain	آلام شديدة في المعدة
Confusion	ارتباك
passing out	فقدان الوعي
inflammation in the veins	التهاب في الأوردة
throbbing or cramping pain, typically in one leg	ألم نابض أو تشنج ، عادة في ساق واحدة
swelling, warmth, and redness in the affected leg	تورم ودفء واحمرار في الساق المصابة
swollen veins that feel hard or sore to the touch	الأوردة المنتفخة التي تشعر بصلابة أو محتقنة مع اللمس
sudden shortness of breath	ضيق مفاجئ في التنفس
chest pain, especially when breathing	ألم في الصدر، خاصة عند التنفس
coughing up blood	السعال أو سعال الدم
irregular heartbeat	اضطراب نبضات القلب
palpitations	خفقان
anxiety	قلق
dizziness, lightheadedness, or fainting	الدوخة أو الدوار أو الإغماء
unexplained leg pain	آلام الساق غير المبررة
swelling in the feet or legs that comes and goes, or that does not get better with time	تورم في القدمين أو الساقين يأتي ويذهب ، أو لا يتحسن مع مرور الوقت
high blood pressure	ضغط دم مرتفع
sudden weakness or numbness only affecting one side of the body	ضعف مفاجئ أو تنميل يؤثر على جانب واحد فقط من الجسم
slurring of speech	التلعثم في الكلام
sudden blindness in one eye	عمى مفاجئ في عين واحدة
Painful cramps on the hips or legs (claudication)	تشنجات مؤلمة في الوركين أو الساقين (العرج)

Erectile dysfunction	الضعف الجنسي لدى الرجال
Breakdown and death of tissue, also known "gangrene"	تلف الأنسجة وموتها ، المعروف أيضًا بالغرغرينا
Coolness or tingling of the foot	برودة أو وخز في القدم
Inability to move the feet	عدم القدرة على تحريك القدمين
Limping	العرج
Sexual intercourse related pain	الآلام المصاحبة في فترة الجماع الجنسي
Pelvic pain	آلام الحوض
Thrombosis/blood clots in veins	تجلط الدم في الأوردة
Thrombosis/blood clots in arteries	تجلط الدم في الشرايين

- **The Common Diseases / Health Conditions**

The Common Diseases / Health Conditions	
Term	المصطلح
Vascular Disorders	اضطرابات الأوعية الدموية
Arteriovenous fistula	ناسور شرياني وريدي
Atherosclerosis	تصلب الشرايين
Chronic venous insufficiency	القصور الوريدي المزمن
Compartment syndrome	متلازمة الحيز
Connective tissue disease	مرض النسيج الضام
Critical limb ischemia	نقص التروية الحرج للأطراف
Deep vein thrombosis (DVT)	الخثار الوريدي العميق
Diabetic foot disease	قدم مريض السكر
Intermittent claudication	العرج المتقطع
Microangiopathy	اعتلال الأوعية الدقيقة
Peripheral artery disease	مرض الشريان المحيطي
Spider vein	تمدد الأوعية الشعيرية, الوريد العنكبوتي
Thrombosis	الخثار
Varicose vein	الدوالي الوريدية
Vascular occlusion/Stenosis	انسداد الأوعية الدموية

Term		المصطلح
Further Disease/health conditions		
Aneurysm -	a bulge or "ballooning" in the wall of an artery	انبعاج أو "انتفاخ" في جدار الشريان	تمدد الأوعية الدموية -
Atherosclerosis -	a disease in which plaque builds up inside your arteries. Plaque is made up of fat, cholesterol, calcium, and other substances found in the blood.	مرض تتراكم فيه اللويحات داخل الشرايين. تتكون البلاك من الدهون والكوليسترول والكالسيوم والمواد الأخرى الموجودة في الدم.	تصلب الشرايين -
Blood Clots, Including Deep Vein Thrombosis And Pulmonary Embolism	is a condition where blood clots form in the deep veins of the legs. Deep vein thrombosis causes a pulmonary embolism when the clots break off, travel up to the lungs and get stuck in the arteries, creating a blockage.	هي حالة تتكون فيها جلطات دموية في الأوردة العميقة للساقين. يسبب تجلط الأوردة العميقة انسدادًا رئويًا عندما تنفصل الجلطات وتنتقل إلى الرئتين وتعلق في الشرايين ، مما يؤدي إلى انسداد.	جلطات الدم ، بما في ذلك تجلط الأوردة العميقة و الانسداد الرئوي
Coronary Artery Disease And Carotid Artery Disease,	diseases that involve the narrowing or blockage of an artery. The cause is usually a buildup of plaque.	الأمراض التي تنطوي على تضيق أو انسداد الشريان. عادة ما يكون السبب هو تراكم البلاك.	مرض الشريان التاجي ومرض الشريان السباتي ،
Raynaud's Disease -	a disorder that causes the blood vessels to narrow when you are cold or feeling stressed	اضطراب يؤدي إلى تضيق الأوعية الدموية عند الشعور بالبرد أو الشعور بالتوتر	مرض رينود -
Stroke -	a serious condition that happens when blood flow to your brain stops.	حالة خطيرة تحدث عندما يتوقف تدفق الدم إلى دماغك.	سكتة دماغية -
Varicose Veins -	swollen, twisted veins that you can see just under the skin	الأوردة المنتفخة الملتوية التي يمكنك رؤيتها تحت الجلد مباشرة	توسع الأوردة – الدوالي
Vasculitis -	inflammation of the blood vessels	التهاب الأوعية الدموية	التهاب الأوعية الدموية -
Abdominal Aortic	are caused by progressive	ناتجة عن ضعف تدريجي في	تمدد الأورطي البطني

English Term	English Description	Arabic Description	Arabic Term
Aneurysms	weakening of the aortic wall creating a "ballooning" of the vessel.	جدار الأبهر مما يؤدي إلى "انتفاخ" الوعاء الدموي.	
Aortic Dissection (AD)	Aortic dissection is the most common catastrophe affecting the aorta. Split in the wall of the artery.	تسلخ الأبهر هو أكثر الكوارث شيوعًا التي تصيب الشريان الأورطي. انقسام في جدار الشريان	تسلخ الشريان الأبهر (الأورطي)
Atherosclerosis	Atherosclerosis is the hardening of the arteries due to a build-up of plaque inside the artery. There are many diseases linked to atherosclerosis.	تصلب الشرايين هو تصلب الشرايين بسبب تراكم الترسبات داخل الشريان. هناك العديد من الأمراض المرتبطة بتصلب الشرايين.	تصلب الشرايين
Buerger's Disease	A rare disorder characterized by inflammation of the small and medium arteries and veins. It affects about 8-11 persons per 100,000 in North America.	اضطراب نادر يتميز بالتهاب الشرايين والأوردة الصغيرة والمتوسطة. يصيب حوالي 8-11 شخصًا لكل 100000 في أمريكا الشمالية.	مرض بورغيرز
Carotid Arteries Disease	Carotid artery disease is defined by the narrowing or blockage of the artery due to plaque build-up.	مرض الشريان السباتي عن طريق تضيق أو انسداد الشريان بسبب تراكم اللويحات.	مرض الشريان السباتي
Chronic Limb-Threatening Ischemia	"Chronic limb-threatening ischemia (CLTI) is a clinical syndrome defined by the presence of peripheral artery disease (PAD) in combination with rest pain, gangrene, or a lower limb ulceration >2 weeks duration. CLTI is associated with amputation, increased mortality and impaired	"الإقفار الذي يهدد الأطراف المزمنة (CLTI) هو متلازمة سريرية يتم تحديدها من خلال وجود مرض الشريان المحيطي (PAD) مع ألم الراحة أو الغرغرينا أو تقرح الطرف السفلي لمدة تزيد عن أسبوعين. يرتبط CLTI بالبتر وزيادة معدل الوفيات وضعف جودة الحياة. . .	الإسكيميا التي تهدد الأطراف المزمنة الإفقار المزمن الذي يهدد الأطراف

English Term	Description	الوصف	المصطلح
	quality of life. . . .		
Chronic Venous Insufficiency (CVS)	Chronic venous insufficiency is a common cause of leg pain and swelling. CVI is also associated with varicose veins.	القصور الوريدي المزمن هو سبب شائع لألم وتورم الساق. يرتبط CVI أيضًا بدوالي الأوردة.	عدم اكتفاء الوريد المزمن (CVI)
Congenital Vascular Malformation	Congenital vascular malformations (CVMs) are growths or birthmarks made up of blood vessels that have not developed correctly.	تشوهات الأوعية الدموية الخلقية (CVMs) هي أورام أو وحمات تتكون من أوعية دموية لم تتطور بشكل صحيح.	تشوه الأوعية الدموية الخلقية
Deep Vein Thrombosis (DVT)	Deep vein thrombosis (DVT) occurs when a blood clot develops in the large veins of the legs or pelvic area. Can also occur in the arm.	يحدث تجلط الأوردة العميقة (DVT) عندما تتطور جلطة دموية في الأوردة الكبيرة في الساقين أو منطقة الحوض.	تخثر الأوردة العميقة (DVT)
Diabetes And Vascular Disease	Diabetes is a disease in the body where blood sugar (glucose) in your body is too high. High blood sugar can increase your risk for vascular disease.	مرض السكري هو مرض يصيب الجسم حيث يكون سكر الدم (الجلوكوز) في الجسم مرتفعًا للغاية. يمكن أن يزيد ارتفاع نسبة السكر في الدم من خطر الإصابة بأمراض الأوعية الدموية.	السكري وأمراض الأوعية الدموية
Fibromuscular Dysplasia	Fibromuscular Dysplasia (FMD) is a medical condition that causes arteries to narrow, enlarge, or tear.	خلل التنسج العضلي الليفي (FMD) هو حالة طبية تسبب تضيق الشرايين أو تضخمها أو تمزقها.	خلل التنسج الليفي العضلي
High Blood Pressure And Vascular Disease	High blood pressure, or hypertension, can cause a lot of damage to the body over time. It increases the risk for life-threatening complications.	يمكن أن يتسبب في ارتفاع ضغط الدم في الكثير من الضرر للجسم بمرور الوقت. يزيد من خطر حدوث مضاعفات تهدد الحياة.	ارتفاع ضغط الدم وأمراض الأوعية الدموية
Kidney Failure And Vascular Disease	The kidneys cleanse the blood of waste products, balance the electrolytes	تنظف الكلى الدم من الفضلات ، وتوازن الشوارد في الجسم ، وتتحكم في ضغط الدم وتحفز	فشل الكلى وأمراض الأوعية الدموية

	in the body, control blood pressure and stimulate the production of red blood cells.	إنتاج خلايا الدم الحمراء.	
Lymphedema	Lymphedema is a common cause of leg or arm swelling due to the collection of too much lymph fluid.	الوذمة الليمفاوية هي سبب شائع لتورم الساق أو الذراع بسبب تجمع الكثير من السوائل الليمفاوية.	ليمفيديما الوذمة الليمفية
Mesenteric Artery Disease (MAD)	Mesenteric artery disease (MAD) is the hardening of the arteries in the blood vessels that supply the body's intestines. Which causes the patient stop eating, causing weight loss.	مرض الشريان المساريقي (MAD) هو تصلب الشرايين في الأوعية الدموية التي تغذي أمعاء الجسم، مما يتسبب في توقف المريض عن الأكل مما يتسبب في فقدان الوزن.	مرض الشرايين الوسطى المساريقي
Peripheral Artery Disease	Peripheral Artery Disease results from a progressive thickening of an artery's lining caused by a buildup of plaque, which narrows or blocks blood flow, reducing the circulation of the blood to a specific organ or region of the body.	ينتج مرض الشريان المحيطي عن سماكة تدريجية لبطانة الشريان ناتجة عن تراكم اللويحات، مما يضيق أو يمنع تدفق الدم، مما يقلل من دوران الدم إلى عضو أو منطقة معينة من الجسم.	مرض الشريان المحيطي
Portal Hypertension	Portal hypertension is high blood pressure of the portal vein. The portal vein, a major vein in the abdomen, collects nutrient-rich blood from the intestines and delivers it to the liver to nourish it, where it is purified for the body to use.	ارتفاع ضغط الدم البابي هو ارتفاع ضغط الدم في الوريد البابي. الوريد البابي، وهو وريد رئيسي في البطن، يجمع الدم الغني بالمغذيات من الأمعاء ويوصله إلى الكبد لتغذيته، حيث يتم تنقيته ليستخدمه الجسم.	ارتفاع ضغط الدم البابي
Post-Thrombotic Syndrome (PTS)	A condition giving rise to pain in the legs (or arms)	حالة تؤدي إلى الشعور بألم في الساقين (أو الذراعين) بعد تاريخ	متلازمة ما بعد التخثر (PTS)

	following a history of a blood clot (DVT)	من الإصابة بجلطة دموية (DVT)	
Pulmonary Embolism (PE)	A pulmonary Embolism (PE) is a blood clot that lodges in the lung arteries. The blood clot forms in the leg, pelvic, or arm veins, then breaks off from the vein wall and travels through the heart into the lung arteries.	الانسداد الرئوي (PE) هو جلطة دموية تستقر في شرايين الرئة. تتشكل الجلطة الدموية في أوردة الساق أو الحوض أو الذراع، ثم تنفصل عن جدار الوريد وتنتقل عبر القلب إلى شرايين الرئة.	الانسداد الرئوي (PE)
Raynaud's Disease	Raynaud's Disease (also called Raynaud's Phenomenon) is a medical condition where the fingers of healthy individuals may become pale in response to severe cold, the effect is exaggerated in those individuals	مرض رينود (يسمى أيضًا ظاهرة رينود) هو حالة طبية حيث قد تصبح أصابع الأفراد الأصحاء شاحبة استجابة للبرد الشديد، ويكون التأثير مبالغًا فيه عند هؤلاء الأفراد	داء رينود
Renovascular Hypertension	High blood pressure caused by the narrowing of the arteries that carry blood to the kidneys	ارتفاع ضغط الدم الناتج عن تضييق الأوعية الدموية الكلوية	ارتفاع ضغط الدم الناتج عن تضيق الأوعية الدموية الكلوية
Stroke	A stroke, or "brain attack," occurs when blood flow to the brain is interrupted by a blood clot or when a blood vessel bursts.	تحدث السكتة الدماغية، أو "النوبة الدماغية"، عندما ينقطع تدفق الدم إلى الدماغ بسبب جلطة دموية أو عندما ينفجر أحد الأوعية الدموية.	سكتة دماغية
Thoracic Aortic Aneurysm (TAA)	Thoracic Aortic Aneurysm (TAA), a disease of the aorta, is the 12th leading cause of death in the United States.	تمدد الأوعية الدموية الأبهري الصدري (TAA)، وهو مرض يصيب الشريان الأورطي، هو السبب الثاني عشر للوفاة في الولايات المتحدة	تمدد الأورطي الصدري (TAA)

English Term	English Definition	Arabic Definition	Arabic Term
Thrombophilia	Thrombophilias can be defined as a group of inherited or acquired disorders that increase a person's risk of developing thrombosis (abnormal "blood clotting") in the veins or arteries.	يمكن تعريف Thrombophilias على أنها مجموعة من الاضطرابات الموروثة أو المكتسبة التي تزيد من خطر إصابة الشخص بتجلط الدم ("تخثر الدم" غير الطبيعي) في الأوردة أو الشرايين.	أهبة التخثر, التهاب الوريد الخثاري
Varicose Veins	Varicose veins are enlarged, bulging superficial veins that can be felt beneath the skin, generally larger than 3-mm in diameter.	تتضخم الدوالي، وتنتفخ الأوردة السطحية التي يمكن الشعور بها تحت الجلد، ويكون قطرها أكبر من 3 مم بشكل عام.	توسع الأوردة (دوالي الأوردة)
Vascular Dementia	Vascular dementia is a condition that causes changes in thinking skills. Vascular dementia can cause problems with memory, speech or balance. Affected by reduced blood flow to the brain.	الخرف الوعائي هو حالة تسبب تغيرات في مهارات التفكير. يمكن أن يسبب الخرف الوعائي مشاكل في الذاكرة أو الكلام أو التوازن. يتأثر بانخفاض تدفق الدم إلى المخ.	الخرف الوعائي
Vasculitis	Vasculitis is an inflammation of the wall of a blood vessel.	التهاب الأوعية الدموية هو التهاب في جدار الوعاء الدموي.	التهاب الأوعية الدموية
Vein Of Galen Malformation (Vogm)	Vein of Galen Malformation (VOGM) is a vascular condition affecting the brain	الوريد من تشوه جالينوس (VOGM)هو حالة الأوعية الدموية التي تؤثر على الدماغ .	عرق تشوه غالين (VOGM)
Spider Veins	Tiny thread-like veins tend mostly on legs which are usually asymptomatic	تميل الأوردة الصغيرة الشبيهة بالخيوط في الغالب على الساقين والتي عادة ما تكون بدون أعراض	عروق العنكبوت
Reticular veins, sometimes called feeder veins or blue veins,	occur when very small veins become dilated which allows the blood to flow backward. This causes the veins to	تحدث عندما تتسع الأوردة مما يسمح للدم بالتدفق للخلف. يؤدي هذا إلى تضخم الأوردة بسبب زيادة الضغط.	الأوردة الشبكية

	enlarge due to the increase in pressure.		
Incompetent veins	Veins which allow blood flow in two directions because of damage to their valves	الأوردة التي تسمح بتدفق الدم في اتجاهين بسبب تلف صماماتها	أوردة لا تعمل بكفاءة
Pelvic congestion syndrome	A condition characterized by abdominal pain due to severely incompetent veins in the abdomen and pelvis	حالة تتميز بألم في البطن بسبب عجز شديد في الأوردة في البطن والحوض	متلازمة احتقان الحوض
Brain hemorrhage	A bleed into the brain	نزيف في المخ	نزيف في المخ
Phlebitis	Inflammation of a vein	التهاب الوريد	الالتهاب الوريدي

Diagnostic Service	المصطلح
Investigations	
Special types of ultrasound technology:	أنواع خاصة من تقنية الموجات فوق الصوتية:
Doppler ultrasound.	الموجات فوق الصوتية دوبلر.
This allows a healthcare provider to see blood flow through arteries and veins. The amount of blood pumped with each heartbeat is a sign of how large a vessel's opening is. A Doppler ultrasound can also find abnormal blood flow in a vessel, which may mean there is a blockage.	يسمح هذا لمقدم الرعاية الصحية برؤية تدفق الدم عبر الشرايين والأوردة. إن كمية الدم التي يتم ضخها مع كل نبضة قلب هي علامة على حجم فتحة الأوعية الدموية. يمكن أن تجد الموجات فوق الصوتية دوبلر أيضًا تدفق دم غير طبيعي في وعاء ، مما قد يعني وجود انسداد.
Color Doppler.	دوبلر ملون.
This is an enhanced form of Doppler ultrasound. It uses different colors to show the direction of blood flow.	هذا شكل محسن من الموجات فوق الصوتية دوبلر. يستخدم ألوانًا مختلفة لإظهار اتجاه تدفق الدم.
Pulse volume recording (PVR) study.	دراسة تسجيل حجم النبض.(PVR).
This is done to assess blood flow in your arms or legs. Blood pressure cuffs are inflated on your arm or leg, and the blood pressure there is measured using the Doppler probe.	يتم إجراء ذلك لتقييم تدفق الدم في ذراعيك أو ساقيك. يتم نفخ كفات ضغط الدم على ذراعك أو رجلك ، ويتم قياس ضغط الدم هناك باستخدام مسبار دوبلر.
Carotid duplex scan.	مسح على الوجهين للشريان السباتي.
This type of Doppler exam checks the carotid arteries in your neck. It gives a 2D (2-dimensional) image of the arteries. This can show the structure of the arteries, the blocked area, and how well blood is flowing.	يفحص هذا النوع من فحص دوبلر الشرايين السباتية في رقبتك. يعطي صورة ثنائية الأبعاد (ثنائية الأبعاد) للشرايين. يمكن أن يوضح هذا بنية الشرايين والمنطقة المسدودة ومدى تدفق الدم.
Carotid artery duplex scan.	مسح مزدوج للشريان السباتي.
This type of vascular ultrasound can check for blockages or narrowing (stenosis) of the carotid arteries in your neck. It can also check the branches of the carotid artery.	يمكن لهذا النوع من الموجات فوق الصوتية للأوعية الدموية أن يفحص انسداد أو تضيق (تضيق) الشرايين السباتية في رقبتك. ويمكنه أيضًا فحص فروع الشريان السباتي.
Angiogram (Angiography)	تصوير الأوعية الدموية
An angiogram is a special X-ray taken as a special dye is injected through a thin, flexible tube called a catheter to detect blockages or aneurysms in blood vessels.	تصوير الأوعية هو أشعة سينية خاصة تؤخذ كصبغة خاصة يتم حقنها من خلال أنبوب رفيع ومرن يسمى قسطرة للكشف عن الانسدادات أو تمدد الأوعية الدموية في الأوعية الدموية.
Computerized tomography (CT) scan	التصوير المقطعي المحوسب(CT)
The cardiac computed tomography scan, or cardiac CT, uses X-rays to create three-dimensional images of your heart and blood vessels.	يستخدم التصوير المقطعي للقلب ، أو التصوير المقطعي المحوسب للقلب ، الأشعة السينية لإنشاء صور ثلاثية الأبعاد للقلب والأوعية الدموية.
Magnetic resonance imaging (MRI)	التصوير بالرنين المغناطيسي (MRI)
Magnetic resonance imaging, better known as cardiac MRI, is a combination of radio waves,	التصوير بالرنين المغناطيسي ، المعروف باسم التصوير بالرنين المغناطيسي للقلب ، هو مزيج من موجات الراديو

magnets, and computer technology to create images of your heart and blood vessels.

والمغناطيس وتكنولوجيا الكمبيوتر لإنشاء صور للقلب والأوعية الدموية.

- Treatment

Treatment	
Term	**المصطلح**
Veins treatment	علاج الأوردة
Endovenous Laser treatment/Ablation of varicose veins (EVLT/EVLA)	العلاج بالليزر داخل الوريد / استئصال الدوالي EVLT / EVLA)
Endovenous Radio Frequency (RF) treatment of varicose veins	العلاج بالترددات الراديوية الوريدية (RF) من الدوالي
Endovenous Glue (Venaseal) treatment of varicose veins	علاج الدوالي الوريدية بالصمغ الوريدي(Venaseal)
Classical surgery for varicose veins (ligation, stripping and phlebotomies)	الجراحة الكلاسيكية لدوالي الأوردة (الربط ، التجريد ، الفصد)
Foam and liquid sclerotherapy of varicose & thread (Spider) veins	المعالجة بالتصليب بالرغوة والسائل للدوالي والخيوط (العنكبوت)
Ultrasound guided foam and liquid sclerotherapy of varicose veins and perforating veins	رغوة موجهة بالموجات فوق الصوتية وعلاج بالتصليب السائل للدوالي والأوردة المثقوبة
Dermal laser therapy of thread, reticular veins and venous malformations Adjuvant & New treatments of varicose veins	العلاج بالليزر الجلدي للخيوط والأوردة الشبكية والتشوهات الوريدية علاجات مساعدة وجديدة للدوالي
Laser & Bi-polar electrotherapy of facial thread veins and telangiectasia	العلاج الكهربائي بالليزر والقطبي الثنائي لأوردة الوجه وتوسع الشعيرات
Superficial venous thrombosis and thrombophlebitis	الخثار الوريدي السطحي والتهاب الوريد الخثاري
Thrombolysis of acute proximal (DVT)	انحلال الخثرة من الداني الحاد(DVT)
Stenting of chronic venous stenoses or occlusions including May-Thurner syndrome	دعامات في حالات التضيق أو الانسداد الوريدي المزمن بما في ذلك متلازمة ماي-ثورنر
Treatment of pulmonary embolism and insertion of IVC filters	علاج الانسداد الرئوي وإدخال فلتر أو مصفاه IVC
Venous bypasses	المجازات الوريدية
Embolization of pelvic varices and venous malformation	إصمام دوالي الحوض والتشوه الوريدي
Treatment of varicocele	علاج دوالي الخصية
Treatment of pelvic congestion syndrome and vulval varices	علاج متلازمة احتقان الحوض ودوالي الصمامات
Treatment of chronic venous leg ulcers and post phlebitis syndrome	علاج تقرحات الساق الوريدية المزمنة ومتلازمة ما بعد التهاب الوريد
Treatment of leg swelling, cellulitis and lymphedema	علاج تورم الساق والتهاب النسيج الخلوي والوذمة اللمفية

Arterial treatment	علاج الشرايين
Treatment of atherosclerosis & intermittent claudication	علاج تصلب الشرايين والعرج المتقطع
Angiograms, angioplasties and vascular stenting	تصوير الأوعية الدموية ورأب الأوعية الدموية والدعامات الوعائية
Surgical and endovascular stenting of abdominal aortic aneurysms	دعامة جراحية وداخل الأوعية الدموية لتمدد الشريان الأورطي البطني
Surgical and endovascular stenting of thoracic aortic aneurysms	دعامة جراحية وداخل الأوعية الدموية لتمدد الأوعية الدموية الأبهري الصدري
Surgical and stenting of limbs aneurysms including femoral, popliteal and subclavian	دعامة جراحية وتمدد الأوعية الدموية في الأطراف بما في ذلك الفخذ والمأبضية وتحت الترقوة
Treatment of carotid artery disease and carotid endarterectomy	علاج مرض الشريان السباتي واستئصال باطنة الشريان السباتي
Arterial bypasses: Ilio-fermoral, femoro-femoral, femoro-popliteal and femoro-distal.	المجازات الشريانية: Ilio-fermoral و -femoro femoral و femoro-popliteal و femoro-distal.
Extra anatomical bypasses: Axillo-femoral, femoro-femoral and obturator foramen bypass	المجازات التشريحية الإضافية: مجازة إبطية - فخذية ، فخذية ـ فخذية ، مجازة سدادة
Embolectomy and/or thrombolysis of acute arterial or bypass occlusions	استئصال الصمة و / أو تخثر الدم من انسداد الشرايين الحاد أو المجازة
Treatment of thoracic outlet syndrome	علاج متلازمة مخرج الصدر
Treatment of arteriovenous malformations & arteriovenous fistulae	علاج التشوهات الشريانية الوريدية والناسور الشرياني الوريدي
Treatment of diabetic foot infections and gangrene	علاج التهابات القدم السكرية والغرغرينا
Treatment of vasoconstrictive disorders (Raynaud's, acrocyanosis & associated conditions)	علاج اضطرابات تضيق الأوعية (رينود ، زراق الأطراف والحالات المرتبطة بها)
Renal & Vascular access service:	**خدمة مداخل الكلى والأوعية الدموية:**
Insertion of dialysis catheters for hemodialysis	إدخال قثاطير لغسيل الدم
Insertion of ports for vascular access and chemotherapy	إدخال منافذ للوصول إلى الأوعية الدموية والعلاج الكيميائي
Insertion of peritoneal dialysis catheters	إدخال قثاطير غسيل الكلى البريتوني
Creation of native arteriovenous fistulae	خلق النواسير الشريانية الوريدية الأصلية
Insertion of PTFE grafts for hemodialysis	إدخال طعوم PTFE لغسيل الكلى
Repair and/or removal of dialysis related implants	إصلاح و / أو إزالة الغرسات المتعلقة بغسيل الكلى
Wound care service & limb salvage unit:	**خدمة العناية بالجروح ووحدة إنقاذ الأطراف:**
Treatment of acute wounds	علاج الجروح الحادة
Treatment of chronic wounds	علاج الجروح المزمنة
Treatment of chronic leg ulcers	علاج تقرحات الساق المزمنة
Treatment of diabetic and vascular gangrene	علاج الغنغرينا السكري و الأوعية الدموية

Treatment of cellulitis	علاج التهاب النسيج الخلوي
Vacuum dressing	ضمادة الفراغ
Nano-technology	تقنية النانو
Prosthetic service:	**خدمة الأطراف الاصطناعية:**
Compression stocking	الجوارب الضاغطة
Compression bandaging	الضمادات الضاغطة
Manual lymphatic drainage (MLD)	التصريف اللمفاوي اليدوي (MLD)
Pressure relief footwear and garments	الملابس والأحذية لتخفيف الضغط
Limb prosthesis	طرف اصطناعي

- Surgery / Procedures

Surgery / Procedures	
Term	المصطلح
Endarterectomy of artery	استئصال باطنة الشريان
a surgery to remove plaque from narrowed or blocked arteries. You may have an endarterectomy to treat peripheral artery disease or carotid artery disease. Your provider makes an incision directly over the blocked artery during the procedure. Then, they use a special tool to remove plaque.	عملية جراحية لإزالة البلاك من الشرايين الضيقة أو المسدودة. قد تخضع لعملية استئصال باطنة الشريان لعلاج مرض الشريان المحيطي أو مرض الشريان السباتي. يقوم مزودك بعمل شق مباشرة فوق الشريان المسدود أثناء العملية. ثم يستخدمون أداة خاصة لإزالة البلاك.
Artery Bypass	جراحة مجازة الشريان
Balloon angioplasty	رأب ترميم الأوردة بالبالون
Stenting	دعامات
is a minimally invasive procedure, meaning it is not considered major surgery. Stents can be made of metal mesh, fabric, silicone, or combinations of materials. Stents used for coronary arteries are made of metal mesh. Fabric stents, also called stent grafts, are used in larger arteries such as the aorta.	هو إجراء طفيف التوغل ، مما يعني أنه لا يعتبر عملية جراحية كبرى. يمكن أن تكون الدعامات مصنوعة من شبكة معدنية أو قماش أو سيليكون أو مزيج من المواد. الدعامات المستخدمة في الشرايين التاجية مصنوعة من شبكة معدنية. تُستخدم الدعامات المصنوعة من القماش ، والتي تسمى أيضًا ترقيع الدعامات ، في الشرايين الكبيرة مثل الشريان الأورطي.
Repair of artery by simple suture	إصلاح الشريان بخياطة بسيطة
Repair of arterioveneous fistula	إصلاح الناسور الشرياني الوريدي
Patch angioplasty using vein graft	تصحيح رأب الوعاء باستخدام طعم الوريد
Repair of abdominal aortic aneurysm	إصلاح تمدد الشريان الأورطي البطني
Carotid endarterectomy	عملية استئصال باطنة الشريان
is a surgical procedure to remove a build-up of fatty deposits (plaque), which cause narrowing of a carotid artery.	هو إجراء جراحي لإزالة تراكم الترسبات الدهنية (اللويحات) ، والتي تسبب تضيق الشريان السباتي.

Vascular trauma	صدمة الأوعية الدموية
occurs when a blood vessel sustains either a blunt injury or a penetrating injury	تحدث عندما يصاب أحد الأوعية الدموية إما بإصابة حادة أو إصابة مخترقة
Embolectomy / thrombectomy	استئصال الصمة / استئصال الخثرة
An embolectomy removes a blood clot that moved from where it started in a blood vessel to another part of your body. a minimally invasive procedure using a catheter or do a traditional surgery.	يزيل استئصال الصمة الجلطة الدموية التي انتقلت من حيث بدأت في الأوعية الدموية إلى جزء آخر من الجسم. إجراء طفيف التوغل باستخدام قسطرة أو إجراء جراحة تقليدية.
Limb amputation:	بتر الأطراف
Amputation is surgery to remove all or part of a limb or extremity (outer limbs)	البتر هو عملية جراحية لإزالة طرف أو طرف أو جزء منه (الأطراف الخارجية)
Lower limb bypass	المجازة للطرف السفلي
Mesenteric bypass	المجازة المساريقية
An aortobifemoral bypass	
is surgery to redirect blood around narrowed or blocked blood vessels in your belly or groin.	هي عملية جراحية لإعادة توجيه الدم حول الأوعية الدموية الضيقة أو المسدودة في البطن أو الفخذ.

Complications	
Term	**المصطلح**
Bleeding	نزيف
Infection	عدوى
Thrombosis	تجلط الدم
Unsuccessful surgery	جراحة غير ناجحة
Embolization	الانصمام, الانسداد
(EM-boh-lih-ZAY-shun) A procedure that uses particles, such as tiny gelatin sponges or beads, to block a blood vessel. Embolization may be used to stop bleeding or to block the flow of blood to a tumor or abnormal area of tissue.	(EM-boh-lih-ZAY-shun) إجراء يستخدم جزيئات ، مثل الإسفنج أو الخرزات الجيلاتينية الصغيرة ، لسد الأوعية الدموية. يمكن استخدام الانصمام لوقف النزيف أو لمنع تدفق الدم إلى الورم أو منطقة غير طبيعية من الأنسجة.
Postoperative pain	ألم ما بعد الجراحة
Swelling	تورم
Peripheral Nerve damage (neuropraxia)	تلف الأعصاب المحيطية (الطرفية)
Non-healing wound	جرح لا يلتئم
Hematoma	ورم دموي
Pulmonary embolization	الانصمام الرئوي
Perforation of other organs	انثقاب الأعضاء الأخرى
Gut ischemia	نقص تروية الأمعاء
Limb loss	فقدان الأطراف
Stroke	السكتة الدماغية
Myocardial infarction	احتشاء عضلة القلب
Reperfusion syndrome	متلازمة ضخة

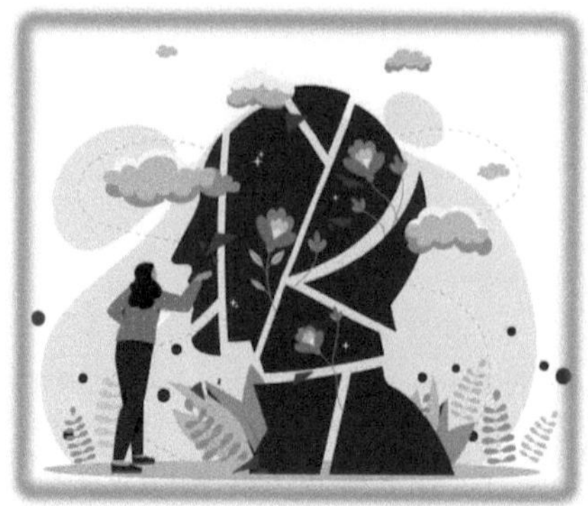

Chapter SEVEN - Neurology & Psychology

Overview

This chapter introduces the reader to common medical terminology of Neurology & Psychology specialty that will include bilingual terminology for the following;

1. Anatomy
2. Common Symptoms of Nervous System Disorder
3. Common Symptoms of Mental / Behavioural / Neurodevelopmental Disorder
4. Common Diseases / Health Conditions
5. Investigations
6. Treatment
7. Surgery / Procedure
8. Complications from diseases/disorders
9. Complications from Medications for Nervous and Mental Health Conditions
10. Neuropsychological Assessment

We hope you enjoy reading this Chapter, and more chapters awaiting you

- **Anatomy**

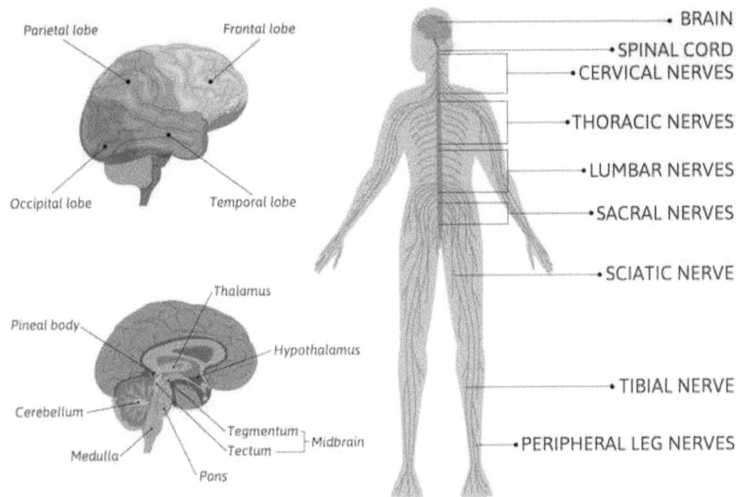

The central nervous system is made up of the brain and spinal cord. The peripheral nervous system consists of the nerves that branch off from the brain and spinal cord and extend to all parts of the body.

الجهاز العصبي المركزي يتكوّن من الدماغ والحبل الشّوكي. الجهاز العصبي المحيطي يتكوّن من الأعصاب المتفرّعة من المخ والحبل الشّوكي والذي يمتدّ إلى كل أجزاء الجسم.

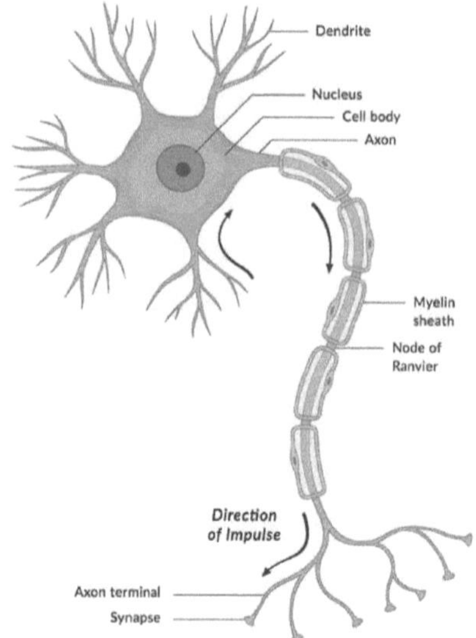

The basic unit of the nervous system is a nerve cell, or **neuron.** The human brain contains about 100 billion neurons. A neuron has a cell body, which includes the cell nucleus, and special extensions called **axons** and **dendrites.** Bundles of axons, called **nerves,** are found throughout the body. Axons and dendrites allow neurons to communicate, even across long distances.

الوحدة الأساسية للجهاز العصبيّ هي **الخليّة العصبيّة أو العصبون.** يحتوي دماغ الإنسان على حوالي 100 مليار خلية عصبية. يحتوي العصبون على جسم خلوي يتضمّن نواة الخليّة، وإمتدادات خاصّة تسمّى **المحاور والتّشعّبات.** جِزَم من المحاور العصبيّة، تسمّى **الأعصاب،** توجد في جميع أرجاء الجسم. تسمح المحاور والتشعبات للخلايا العصبية بالتواصل، حتى عبر مسافات طويلة.

Different types of neurons control or perform different functions. For instance, **motor neurons** transmit signals from the brain to the muscles to generate movement. **Receptors** that detect light, sound, odor, taste, pressure, and heat; trigger nerve impulses in **sensory neurons** that send those impulses to the brain. Other parts of the nervous system control involuntary functions. These include keeping a regular heartbeat, releasing hormones, controlling the pupil in response to light, and regulating the digestive system.

أنواع مختلفة من الخلايا العصبية تتحكم أو تؤدّي وظائف مختلفة. على سبيل المثال، تُنقل **الخلايا العصبية الحركية** الإشارات من الدِّماغ إلى العضلات لتوليد الحركة. **مستقبلات** تستشعر الضوء، الصوت، الرّائحة، التّذوُّق، الضغط والحرارة؛ تُحفِّز دوافع عصبية فى **الخلايا العصبية الحسيّة** والتي تنقل هذه الإشارات إلى الدماغ. أجزاء أخرى من الجهاز العصبي تتحكم بالوظائف اللاإرادية. وتشمل هذه الحفاظ على نبضات القلب المنتظمة، إفراز الهرمونات، التحكم ببؤبؤ العين إستجابةً للضوء، وتنظيم الجهاز الهضمي.

When a neuron sends a signal to another neuron, it sends an electrical signal down the length of its axon via an **action potential** generated by the flow of Sodium, Potassium and Calcium ions through channels across the membrane. At the end of the axon, the electrical signal changes to a chemical signal by releasing **neurotransmitters** into the **synapse** —the space between the end of an axon and the tip of a dendrite from another neuron.

عندما تُرسل عصبون إشارة إلى عصبون آخر، فإنها تُرسل إشارة كهربائية على طول محورها من خلال **السيال العصبي** التي ينتجها حركة آيونات الصوديوم و البوتاسيوم و الكالسيوم عبر القنوات في الغشاء العصبي. عند نهاية المحور العصبي، تتحوّل الإشارة الكهربائية إلى إشارة كيميائية **بإفراز ناقلات عصبية** إلى المِشبك العصبي – المساحة بين نهاية محور عصبون وطرف تشعبات عصبون آخر.

The nervous system also includes non-neuron cells, called **glia** (pronounced *GLEE-ah*). Glia perform many important functions that keep the nervous system working properly. They help support and hold neurons in place, protect neurons, create insulation called **myelin sheath** which helps move nerve impulses, repair neurons and help restore neuron function, remove dead neurons and regulate neurotransmitters.

يحتوي الجهاز العصبي أيضاً على خلايا غير عصبية تُسمى **خلايا رابطة أو خلايا دِبْقيّة.** تؤدي الخلايا الدِّبقية وظائف مهمة عديدة والتي تحافظ على عمل الجهاز العصبي بشكل صحيح. إنها تساعد في دعم والمحافظة على الخلايا العصبية في مكانها، وتحميها، وتُكوّن صفيحة عازلة تسمى **غمد الميلين أو غشاء الميلين** والتي تساعد في تحسين حركة الإشارات الكهربائية، وتساعد في إصلاح العصبونات واستعادة وظيفتها، إزالة الأعصاب الميّتة، وتنظيم الناقلات العصبية.

The brain is made up of many networks of communicating neurons and glia that work together to control body functions, emotions, thinking, behavior, and other activities. The human brain is basically symmetrical, split down the middle: the *right* cerebral hemisphere receives sensory input from and directs movement on the *left side* of the body, while the *left* hemisphere governs corresponding functions for the *right side*.

تتكون الدماغ من شبكات تواصل كثيرة بين الخلايا العصبية والخلايا الدبقية التي تعمل معاً للتحكم بوظائف جسدية، والعواطف، والتفكير، والسلوك، ووظائف أخرى. إن الدماغ البشري

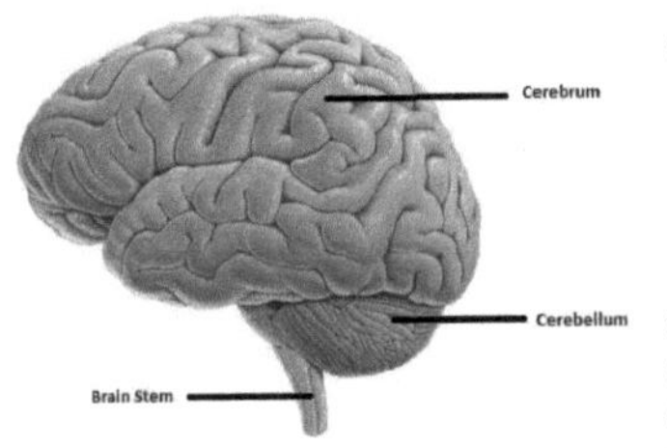

The three main parts of the brain are the **cerebrum, cerebellum** and **brain stem.**

للدماغ ثلاثة أجزاء رئيسية هي **المخ، المخيخ وجذع الدماغ**

أو **النخاع المستطيل.**

The largest part of the brain, the **cerebrum,** initiates and coordinates movement and regulates temperature. Other areas of the cerebrum enable speech, judgment, thinking and reasoning, problem-solving, emotions and learning. Other functions relate to vision, hearing, touch, and other senses.

المخ هو الجزء الأكبر من الدماغ، يتحكّم بإنشاء وتنسيق الحركة وتنظيم درجة الحرارة الجسم. وهناك مناطق أخرى في المخ تُمكّن التحدّث والإحكام والتفكير والاستدلال، وحل المشاكل، والعواطف والتّعلّم. ووظائف أخرى تتعلّق بالرّؤية والسّمع واللّمس وحواس أخرى.

The cerebellum ("little brain") is a fist-sized portion of the brain located at the back of the head, and above the brainstem. Its function is to coordinate voluntary muscle movements and to maintain posture, balance, and equilibrium. New studies are exploring the cerebellum's roles in thought, emotions, and social behavior, as well as its possible involvement in addiction, autism and schizophrenia.

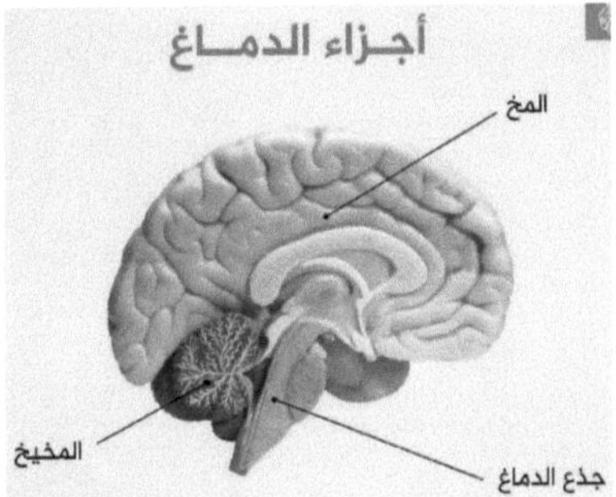

المخيخ بحجم قبضة اليد وموقعه في مؤخرة الرأس، فوق جذع الدماغ. وظيفته تنسيق حركة العضلات الإرادية والمحافظة على وضعية الجسم والتوازن وإعادة الاتزان. هناك دراسات جديدة تستكشف دور المخيخ في التفكير و العواطف والسلوك الاجتماعي، وتورطه المحتمل في الإدمان والتّوحّد وانفصام الشخصية.

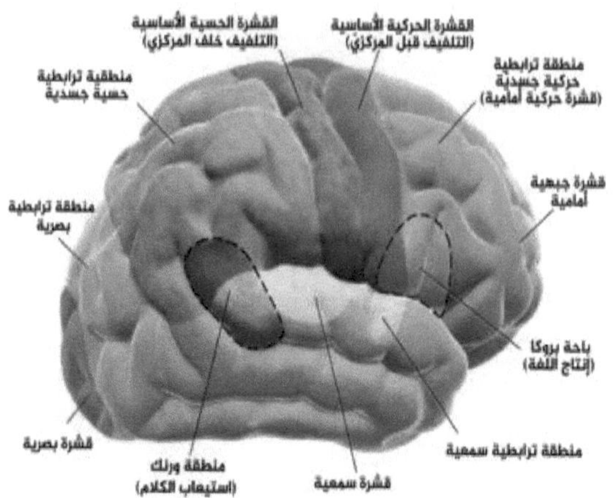

القشرة الحسية الأساسية (التلفيف خلف المركزي)
القشرة الحركية الأساسية (التلفيف قبل المركزي)
منطقة ترابطية حسية جسدية
منطقة ترابطية حركية جسدية (قشرة حركية أمامية)
منطقة ترابطية بصرية
قشرة جبهية أمامية
قشرة بصرية
باحة بروكا (إنتاج اللغة)
منطقة ورنك (استيعاب الكلام)
قشرة سمعية
منطقة ترابطية سمعية

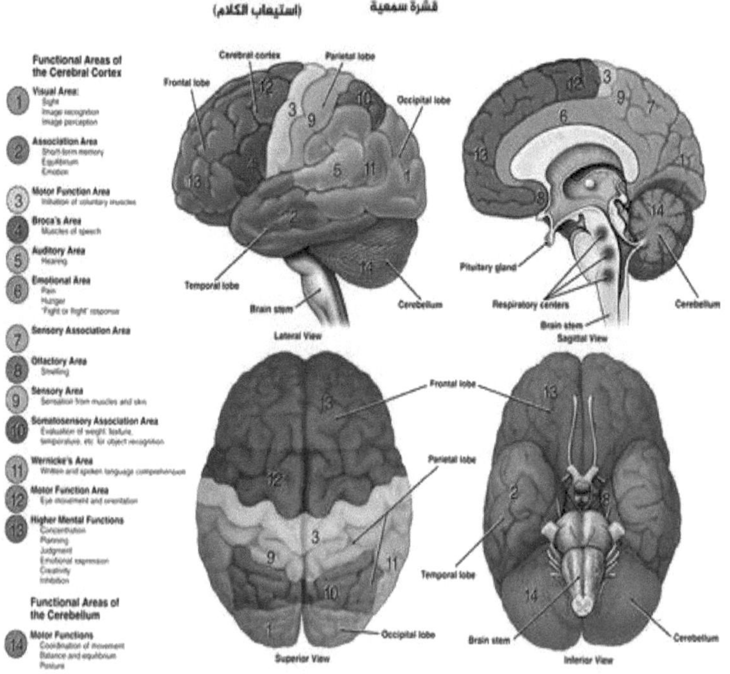

Functional Areas of the Cerebral Cortex
1 Visual Area:
Sight
Image recognition
Image perception
2 Association Area
Short-term memory
Equilibrium
Emotion
3 Motor Function Area
Initiation of voluntary muscles
4 Broca's Area
Muscles of speech
5 Auditory Area
Hearing
6 Emotional Area
Pain
Hunger
'Fight or flight' response
7 Sensory Association Area
8 Olfactory Area
Smelling
9 Sensory Area
Sensation from muscles and skin
10 Somatosensory Association Area
Evaluation of weight, texture,
temperature, etc. for object recognition
11 Wernicke's Area
Written and spoken language comprehension
12 Motor Function Area
Eye movement and orientation
13 Higher Mental Functions
Concentration
Planning
Judgment
Emotional expression
Creativity
Inhibition
Functional Areas of the Cerebellum
14 Motor Functions
Coordination of movement
Balance and equilibrium
Posture

Cerebral cortex
Parietal lobe
Frontal lobe
Occipital lobe
Temporal lobe
Brain stem
Cerebellum
Lateral View

Pituitary gland
Respiratory centers
Brain stem
Cerebellum
Sagittal View

Frontal lobe
Parietal lobe
Temporal lobe
Occipital lobe
Superior View

Frontal lobe
Parietal lobe
Temporal lobe
Brain stem
Cerebellum
Inferior View

NERVOUS SYSTEM

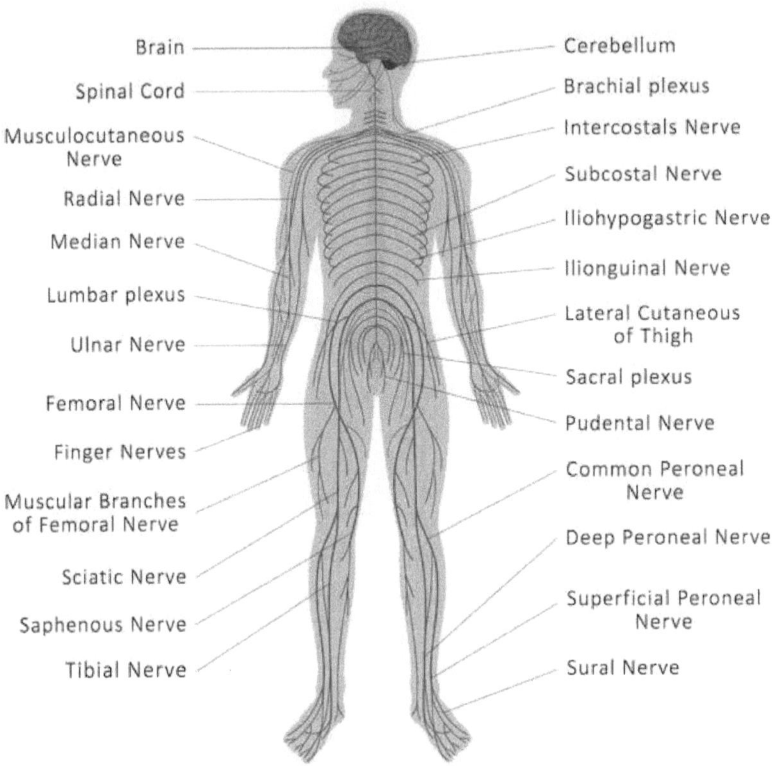

المناطق الوظيفية للقشرة الدماغية

① **منطقة البصر**
الرؤية
التعرف على الصور
إدراك الصورة

② **منطقة الترابط**
الذاكرة قصيرة الأمد
التوازن
المشاعر

③ **منطقة وظيفة الحركة**
تنشيط العضلات الإرادية

④ **منطقة بروكا**
العضلات اللازمة للتحدث

⑤ **منطقة السمع**
السمع

⑥ **منطقة العاطفة**
الألم
الجوع
إستجابة "الكر والفر"

⑦ **منطقة الروابط الحسية**

⑧ **منطقة حاسة الشم**
الشّم

⑨ **منطقة الحسية**
الأحاسيس من العضلات والجلد

⑩ **منطقة الترابط الجسدي الحسّي**
تقييم الوزن، الملمس، درجة الحرارة، الخ، للتّعرّف على الأشياء

⑪ **منطقة فرنيك**
إستيعاب اللغة المنطوقة والمكتوبة

⑫ **منطقة الوظائف الحركية**
حركة العينين والتوجيه

⑬ **وظائف عقلية العليا**
التركيز
التخطيط
الإحكام
التعبير العاطفي
الإبداع
التثبيط

المناطق الوظيفية في المخيخ
⑭ **الوظائف الحركية**
تنسيق الحركة
التوازن وإعادة الإتزان
وضعية الجسم

- **The Common Symptoms of Nervous System disorder**

The Common Symptoms	
Term	المصطلح
Numbness	خدران /تنمّل
Tingling	وخز
Loss of sensation	فقدان الإحساس
Persistent headache	صداع مستديم
Sudden onset headache	صداع مفاجئ
Headache that changes	صداع يتغير
Increased sensitivity to light "eye discomfort in bright light" "Photophobia"	زيادة الحساسية للضوء
Increased sensitivity to sound or "a persistent, abnormal, and unwarranted fear of sound" "Phonophobia"	زيادة الحساسية للصوت
Increased sensitivity to smell "Hyperosmia"	زيادة الحساسية للرائحة
Visual aura	هالة بصرية
Weakness/ Loss of muscle strength	ضعف أو وهن/ فقدان قوة العضلات
Muscle wasting "Muscle atrophy" is the thinning of the muscle	هُزال عضلي
Muscular dystrophy "abnormal function of muscle" is muscle disease.	ضمور وخَثَل العضلات
Stiffness/ Muscle rigidity	جمود, تيبس
Spasm	تشنج
Tremors	رُعاش
Convulsive seizures	صرعات أو نوبات تشنّجية
Non-convulsive seizures	صرعات أو نوبات بدون تشنّج
Absence seizures	نوبات صرعية مصحوبة بغيبات الوعي
Dizziness	دوخة
Vertigo	دوار
Double vision	رؤية مزدوجة
Blindness/ Loss of vision	عمى / فقدان البصر
Lack of coordination "ataxia"	نقص التنسيق" الرنح/الاختلاج الحركيّ"
Memory loss	فقدان الذاكرة
Cognitive impairment	الضّعف الإدراكيّ
Behavioural/Personality changes	تغيرات سلوكية/ شخصيّة
Imbalance	عدم توازن
Back pain radiating to lower extremities	آلام الظهر تمتد إلى الأطراف السفلية

Neck pain radiating to upper extremities	ألم الرقبة يمتد إلى الأطراف العلوية
Slurred speech "unclear speech"	كلام غير واضح
Dysarthria (pronounced "dis-AR-three-uh") is a motor speech disorder that makes it difficult to form and pronounce words.	"عّسر التلفظ" أو "صعوبة النطق" أو "عسر الكلام" هو اضطراب الكلام الحركي الذي يجعل من الصعب تكوين الكلمات ونطقها.
Aphasia "meaningless words or speech" is a language disorder caused by damage in a specific area of the brain that controls language expression and comprehension.	الحبسة "احتباس الكلام" هي اضطراب لغوي ناتج عن تلف منطقة معينة من الدماغ تتحكم في التعبير والفهم اللغوي.
Dysphasia "incomplete meaningless words or speech" is a language disorder that affects how you speak and understand language.	عسر التعبير الكلام هو اضطراب لغوي يؤثر على طريقة تحدثك وفهمك للغة

- **The Common Symptoms of Mental / Behavoiural / Neurodevelopmental Disorder**

The Common Symptoms of Mental / Behavoiural / Neurodevelopmental Disorder	
Term	المصطلح
Constant sadness	حزن مستمر
Irritability	حِدّة المزاج
Constant fatigue	إجهاد مستمر
Changes in eating patterns	تغيرات في نمط التغذية
Changes in sleeping patterns	تغيرات في نمط النوم
Difficulty concentrating	صعوبة في التركيز
Confused thinking	تفكير مشوش
Extreme mood changes	تغيرات شديدة في المزاج
Excessive fears or worries	مخاوف أو قلق مفرط
Extreme feelings of guilt	إحساس شديد بالذنب
Withdrawal from friends and family	الانسحاب من الأهل والأصدقاء
Loss of enthusiasm for activities that used to provide pleasure	فقدان الحماس للأنشطة التي كانت ممتعة في السابق
Inability to cope with daily stress	عدم القدرة على التعامل مع الضغوط اليومية
Trouble relating to situations or people	صعوبة في الترابط بالمواقف أو الأشخاص
Detachment from reality/ Delusions	الإنفصال عن الواقع/ الأوهام
Hallucinations "visual, auditory"	الهلوسة "البصرية والسمعية"
Paranoia	جنون الإضطهاد
Psychosis	ذُهان/ إضطراب عقلي
Substance misuse	شرب وتعاطي الكحوليات أو المخدرات
Sexual dysfunction	العجز الجنسي
Excessive anger/ hostility	غضب مفرط/ عدائية
Suicidal thoughts/ ideation	أفكار إنتحارية
Constant thoughts about death	أفكار مستمرة عن الموت
Headaches or body aches with no specific cause	صداع أو أوجاع بالجسم بدون سبب معيّن
Flashbacks	ومضة ذكريات الماضي
Hypervigilance	اليقظة المفرطة
Intrusive memories	ذكريات متطفلة
Nightmares	الكوابيس

The Common Disease/health conditions	
Acute spinal cord injury	إصابة حادّة بالنخاع الشوكي
Arnold–Chiari malformation Disease	تشوه آرنولد – كياري
Dementia is not a specific disease but is rather a general term for the impaired ability to remember or think or make decisions, and this interferes with doing everyday activities.	الخرف / الإعتلال العقليّ ليس مرضاً محدّداً ولكنه مصطلح عام يشير إلى ضعف القدرة على التَّذكّر أو التَّفكير أو إتخاذ القرارات ، والتي يتداخل مع القيام بالأنشطة اليوميّة.
Alzheimer's disease	مرض النسيان، مرض الزهايمر
Vascular dementia	الخرف الوعائي
Lewy body dementia	خرف أجسام ليوي، داء جسيمات ليوي
Frontotemporal dementia "Frontotemporal disorders (FTD)"	الخرف الجبهي الصدغي
Cerebral palsy	الشلل الدماغي
Multiple sclerosis	التَّصلّب العصبيّ المتعدّد
Brain tumours	أورام المخ
Migraine headache	صداع النصفي / شقيقة
Cerebral aneurism	تمدد الأوعية الدَّمويّة الدِّماغية
Amyotrophic Lateral Sclerosis (ALS)	التصلب الجانبي الضموري
Chiari malformation	تشوّه كِياري
Cluster headaches	الصداع العنقودي
Dystonia is a neurological movement disorder characterized by involuntary (unintended) muscle contractions that cause slow repetitive movements or abnormal postures that can sometimes be painful.	خلل التوتر العضلي هو اضطراب حركي عصبي يتميز بانقباضات عضلية لا إرادية (غير مقصودة) تسبب حركات بطيئة متكررة أو أوضاع غير طبيعية يمكن أن تكون مؤلمة في بعض الأحيان.
Encephalitis is the inflammation of brain tissue	إلتهاب الدِّماغ
Meningitis is an inflammation/infection of the protective membranes covering the brain and spinal cord.	إلتهاب السَّحايا/ الحمَّى الشوكية هو التهاب/عدوى في الأغشية الواقية التي تغطي الدماغ والحبل الشوكي.
Epilepsy and seizures	الصَّرع والنَّوبات
Head injury	إصابة بالرَّأس
Peripheral Neuropathy refers to many conditions that involve damage to the peripheral nervous system.	إعتلال الأعصاب الطَّرفيّة يشير ألى العديد من الحالات التي تنطوي على تلف الجهاز العصبيّ المحيطي.
Guillain-Barre Syndrome/ acute inflammatory demyelinating polyneuropathy	متلازمة غيان-باريه / إلتهاب الجذور والأعصاب الحاد المجهول السبب
Carpal tunnel syndrome	متلازمة النفق الرسغي
Bell's palsy	شلل العصب الوجهي/ شلل بيل
Restless leg syndrome	متلازمة تململ الساق

Parkinson's disease	الشّلَل الرُّعاشي / مرض باركِنْسُن
Narcolepsy is a chronic neurological disorder that affects the brain's ability to control sleep-wake cycles	الخدار" النوم القهري" هو اضطراب عصبي مزمن يؤثر على قدرة الدماغ على التحكم في دورات النوم والاستيقاظ
Normal pressure hydrocephalus	استسقاء الرأس ذو الضغط الطبيعي
Hydrocephalus	مَوَه الرّأس / تضخّم الرّأس
Neurocutaneous syndromes are disorders that affect the brain, spinal cord, organs, skin and bones.	المتلازمات العصبيّة الجلديّة هي إضطرابات تؤثر على الدّماغ والحبل الشّوكيّ والأعضاء والجِلد والعظام.
Neurofibromatosis	الورم العصبيّ اللّيفيّ
Tuberous Sclerosis Complex	التّصلّب الدّرني المُعقّد / التّصلّب الحدبيّ المُعقّد
Stroke	سكتة دماغية
Shingles	قوباء منطقية
Paraneoplastic syndromes are a group of rare disorders that occur when the immune system has a reaction to a tumour.	متلازمات الأباعد الورمية هي مجموعة من الاضطرابات النادرة التي تحدث عندما يتفاعل الجهاز المناعي مع ورم
Post-operative syndrome	متلازمة ما بعد العملية
Myasthenia Gravis	الوهن العضليّ الوخيم
Tourette Syndrome (TS) is a condition of the nervous system that causes people to have "tics". Tics are sudden twitches, movements, or sounds that people do repeatedly.	متلازمة توريت (TS) هي حالة تصيب الجهاز العصبي يسبب للناس "التشنجات اللاإرادية". التشنجات اللاإرادية هي تشنجات مفاجئة أو حركات أو أصوات يفعلها الناس بشكل متكرر.
Trigeminal neuralgia (TN), also known as (tic douloureux), or fifth cranial nerve, is a type of chronic pain disorder that involves sudden, severe facial pain.	ألم العصب الثلاثي التوائم (TN) ، المعروف أيضًا باسم تيك دولورو ، أو آلام العصب القحفي الخامسهو نوع من اضطرابات الألم المزمن التي تتضمن ألمًا مفاجئًا وشديدًا في الوجه.
Vasculitis in the brain is inflammation of blood vessels in the brain.	التهاب الأوعية الدموية في الدماغ.
Feeding and Eating disorders	اضطرابات التغذية والأكل
Anorexia nervosa	فقدان الشهية العصبي
Bulimia nervosa	نُهامٌ عُصابيّ
Neurodevelopmental disorders	اضطرابات النمو العصبي
Attention Deficit Hyperactivity disorder (ADHD)	اضطرابات نقص الإنتباه وفرط النشاط
Autism Spectrum disorder	اضطراب ذاتويّ / التّوحّد
Mood disorders	اضطرابات المزاج
Depression disorders	اضطرابات الإكتئاب
Post-partum depression is a type of depression	إكتئاب ما بعد الولادة
Bipolar disorders; formerly called Manic Depressive disorder.	اضطراب ثنائي القطب المعروف سابقاً باضطراب الهوس الاكتئابي
Premenstrual dysphoric disorder	اضطراب ما قبل الحيض/ اضطراب ما قبل الطّمث

	الإكتئابي
Anxiety or fear-related disorders	القلق أو الاضطرابات المرتبطة بالخوف
Panic disorder	اضطراب الهلع
Post-Traumatic Stress disorder	اضْطِرابُ الكَرْبِ التَّالي للرَّضْح
Generalized Anxiety disorder	اضْطِرابُ القَلَق المُتَعَمِّم
Obsessive Compulsive disorder	للوسواس القهرى
Phobias	الرّهاب
Separation anxiety	اضطراب قلق الانفصال
Social anxiety	القلق الاجتماعي
Schizophrenia Spectrum and other psychotic disorders	طيف الفُصام والإضطرابات الذهنيّة الأخرى
Schizophrenia	الفُصام
Delusional Disorder	اضطراب الوهم/ اضطراب توهّم
Schizoaffective disorder is a combination of Schizophrenia and a mood disorder	اضْطِرابٌ فُصاميٌّ عاطِفيّ هو مزيج من الفُصام واضطراب مِزاجيّ.
Post-partum Psychosis; a rare and severe mental health emergency related to post-partum depression	ذهان ما بعد الولادة هي حالة صحيّة عقليّة طارئة، نادرة و شديدة، مرتبطة بالإكتئاب ما بعد الولادة.
Substance/medication-induced psychotic disorder	اضطراب ذهانيّ ناتج عن تعاطي المخدّرات أو الدواء
Behavioural disorders	اضطرابات سُلوكيّة
Conduct disorder	اضطراب السلوك
Oppositional Defiant disorder	اضطراب التَّحدي المُعارِض/ اضطراب العِناد الشّارد
Personality Disorders	
Antisocial Personality Disorder	اضطراب الشّخصيّة المُعادية للمجتمع
Narcissistic Personality Disorder	اضطراب الشّخصيّة النّرجسيّة
Avoidant Personality Disorder	اضطراب الشّخصيّة التَّجنُّبيّة/ اضطراب الشّخصيّة الإنطوائيّة
Dependent Personality Disorder	اضطراب الشّخصيّة الإعتِماديّة
Paranoid Personality Disorder	اضطراب الشّخصيّة المُرتابة/ اضطراب الشّخصيّة الزوراني
Schizoid Personality Disorder	اضطراب الشّخصيّة شبه الفُصامي
Brain tumors	أورام الدماغ

Investigations of Neurological & Mental/ Behavioural/ Neurodevelopmental Disorders	
Diagnostic Service	المصطلح
CT scan	أشعة مقطعية
Electroencephalogram (EEG)	مخطط كهربائي للدماغ
MRI "Magnetic resonance imaging"	التصوير بالرنين المغناطيسي
Electromyography (EMG)	تخطيط العضلات الكهربائي
Nerve Conduction Velocity (NCV)	سرعة التوصيل العصبي
Positron Emission Tomography (PET)	تصوير مقطعي بإطلاق البوزيترون
Arteriogram/ Angiogram	تخطيط الشريان/ مخطط الأوعية الدموية
Spinal tap/ Lumbar puncture	بَزْلٌ قَطنِيّ / ثقب قطني
Evoked potentials	الجُهْدُ المُحَرَّض
Myelogram	مُخَطّط النُّخَاع العَظْمِيّ
Neurosonography or Brain sonography	التصوير بالموجات فوق الصوتية للدماغ
Carotid ultrasound	الموجات فوق الصوتية للشرايين السباتية
Transcranial Doppler	الدوبلر عبر الجمجمة
Ultrasound/ Sonography	صوير بالموجات فوق صوتية / تخطيط صوتي
Electronystagmography	تَخطيطُ كَهرَبِيّة الرَأرَأة
Polysomnogram or Sleep study	اختبارات النوم المتعددة أو إختبار النوم
Biopsy	خُزعة
Dopamine transporter scan (DaT scan) is a diagnostic method that uses a radiopharmaceutical called Ioflupane to measure the function of dopamine transporters (DaT) in the brain. Used to differentiate between movement disorders.	DaTSCAN هي طريقة تشخيصية تستخدم مركبا صيدلانيا إشعاعيا يسمى Ioflupane لقياس وظيفة ناقلات الدوبامين (DaT) في الدماغ. يستخدم للتمييز بين اضطرابات الحركة.
Full health evaluation	تقييم صحي كامل
Blood workup	فحوصات دم
Neurological tests	فحوصات الأعصاب
Mental Health assessment	تقييم الصحة النفسية
Urine tests	فحص البول
Thyroid function test	اختبار وظائف الغدة الدرقية
Test for Anaemia	إختبار لفقر الدّم
B12 deficiency test	اختبار نقص فيتامين B12
Neuropsychological assessment	التقييم العصبي النفسي

- Treatment

Term	المصطلح
Acceptance and Commitment Therapy (ACT)	علاج القبول والإلتزام
Antidepressants such as Selective Serotonin Reuptake Inhibitors (SSRIs)	مضادات الأكتئاب مثل مُثَبِّطَات انْتِقَائِيَّة لإعَادَة الْتِقَاط السِّيرُوتُونِين
Antipsychotics	مضادات الذهان
Antianxiety drugs	دَواءٌ مُضادٌ للقَلَق
Antiepileptics	مضاد صرع
Antiplatelets	مُضَادُّ الصُّفيِحات
Anti-inflammatories	مضاد للالتهابات
Anticoagulants	مضادات التَخثر
Cognitive Behavioural Therapy (CBT)	العلاج السلوكي المعرفي
Dialectical Behavioural Therapy (DBT)	العلاج السلوكي الجدلي
Drug pumps	مضخة توصيل الدواء
Electroconvulsive therapy	العلاج بالصدمات الكهربائية
Family Therapy	لعلاج الأسري
Group therapy	العلاج الجماعيّ
Hypnotherapy	المُعالَجَةَ بالتَّنويِم
Individual therapy	العلاج الفردي
Interpersonal therapy	العلاج التفاعلي
Marital therapy	علاج زواجي
Medications	أدوية
Mood stabilizers	مثبتات المزاج
Neurorehabilitation	إعادة التأهيل العصبي
Occupational therapy	العلاج الوظيفي أو العلاج المهني
Psychotherapy	المُعالَجَةَ النَّفْسِيَّة
Physical Therapy/ Rehabilitation	العلاج الطبيعي / إعادة تأهيل
Psychodynamic Psychotherapy	العلاج النفسي الديناميكي
Repetitive transcranial magnetic stimulation	التحفيز المغناطيسي عبر الجمجمة
Supportive Psychotherapy	المُعالَجَةَ النَّفْسِيَّةَ الدَّاعِمَة
Speech and Language therapy	علاج النطق واللغة
Spinal Cord Stimulation	تحفيز الحبل الشوكي
Stimulation Therapies	علاجات تحفيزية
Vagus nerve stimulation	تحفيز العصب المبهم

Surgery / Procedures	
Term	المصطلح
Deep Brain Stimulation	التحفيز العميق للدماغ
Brain surgery	جراحة الدماغ
Craniotomy (Cranictomy incision)	حَجُّ القِحْف
Burr Hole Procedure	إجراء ثَقب في غلاف المخ
Chiari decompression	تخفيف الضغط الكياري
Spine surgery	جراحة العمود الفقري

- ## Complications from diseases / disorders

Complications of Neurological, Mental, Behavioural, Neurodevelopmental Diseases and Disorders	
Term	المصطلح
Learning difficulties	صعوبات التعلم
Aspiration pneumonia	الالتهاب الرئوي الشفطي
Injury from falls, self-inflicted bites, operating machinery or driving during seizure attack	إصابات بسبب السقوط، أو عضّات ذاتيّة، أو تشغيل آلات أو القيادة أثناء حدوث نوبة صرع
Permanent Brain damage	ضرر دائم في الدماغ
Sudden Unexpected Death in Epilepsy (SUDEP)	الموت المفاجئ غير المتوقع في الصرع
Stroke	سكتة دماغية
Brain edema	وذمة الدماغ
Pneumonia	الالتهاب الرئوي
Aphasia "meaningless words or speech": is a language disorder caused by damage in a specific area of the brain that controls language expression and comprehension.	الحبسة "احتباس الكلام": هي اضطراب لغوي ناتج عن تلف منطقة معينة من الدماغ تتحكم في التعبير والفهم اللغوي.
Slurred speech "unclear speech" Dysarthria (pronounced "dis-AR-three-uh") is a motor speech disorder that makes it difficult to form and pronounce words.	"عُسر التلفظ" "صعوبة النطق" كلام غير واضح "كلام غير واضح" "عسر الكلام" عسر الكلام هو اضطراب الكلام الحركي الذي يجعل من الصعب تكوين الكلمات ونطقها.
Seizures	نوبات / صرعات
UTI and/or bladder control problems	عدوى المسالك البولية أو/مع مشاكل بالتحكم في المثانة
Deep vein thrombosis	تجلط الأوردة العميقة
Clinical depression	الاكتئاب
Physical and/or mental dysfunction	خلل جسدي أو/مع خلل عقلي
Limb contracture	تقلص الأطراف تَقَفُّعُ الأطراف
Weakness	ضعف
Spasticity	تشنج
Shingles	القوباء المنطقية
Post-herpetic neuralgia (PHN)	الألَمُ العَصَبِيُّ التَّالي للهَرْيس
Eye problems including blindness	مشاكل العين بما في ذلك العمى
Pneumonia	الالتهاب الرئوي
Hearing problems	مشاكل السمع
Encephalitis	التهابُ الدّماغ
Death	الموت، منية؛ ميتَة؛ وفاة
Headache, neck pain	صداع، ألم بالرقبة
Hearing or balance problems, tinnitus	مشاكل السمع أو التوازن، الطنين

Dizziness, vomiting	الدَّوار أو الدَّوخة، التقيؤ
Muscle weakness, numbness, hand coordination problems	ضعف العضلات، تنميل، مشاكل بالتنسيق اليدوي
Difficulty swallowing, speaking, breathing	صعوبة في البلع، التحدّث، التنفّس
Insomnia	الأرق
Guillaine-Barre Syndrome	مُتَلازِمَةَ غِيَّان باريه
Gradually increasing weakness in limbs and face	ضعف تدريجي في الأطراف والوجه
Speaking and swallowing difficulties	صعوبة في التحدث والبلع
Death due to paralysis of breathing muscles, septicemia, pulmonary embolism or cardiac arrest	الوفاة بسبب شلل عضلات التنفس أو تسمم الدم أو الانسداد الرئوي أو السكتة القلبية
Ataxia	تَهَزُّع أو إختلال الحركة
Dizziness	دوخة أو دوران
Spasticity, Rigidity	الشلل التشنجي، تَجَمُّد
Tremor	ارتعاش أو رجفة
Orthostatic hypotension	نَقْصُ ضَغْطِ الدَّمِ الإنْتِصابِيّ
Bowel or bladder dysfunction	إختلال بوظائف المثانة و الأمعاء
Sexual dysfunction	إختلال الوظيفة الجنسية
Depression	الاكتئاب
Falls	السقوط، الوقوع
Aspiration pneumonia	الْتِهابٌ رِئَوِيٌّ شَفْطِيّ
Restlessness/sleeplessness	التَّمَلْمُل/ الأرق
Wandering	تجوّل، هائم
Malnutrition, dehydration	سُوءُ التَّغْذِيَة، جفاف
Dementia	خَرَف
Memory loss	فقدان الذّاكرة
Psychological changes	تغيرات نفسية
Cognitive deficits	العجز الإدراكي
Headaches	صداع
Fatigue	إجهاد عصبيّ أو تعب
Nausea	غثيان
Vomiting	القيء
Numbness	تنميل

- **Complications from medications for Neurology or Mental Health Diseases & disorders**

Complications from medications for Neurology or Mental Health Diseases and disorders	
Term	المصطلح
Amyloid-related Imaging Abnormalities (ARIA)	تشوهات التصوير المرتبطة بالعلاج بالأميلويد
Allergic reactions	رد فعل تحسّسي
Temporary swelling in areas of the brain	تورم مؤقت في مناطق الدماغ
Dizziness, Nausea, vomiting	دوخة أو دوران، غثيان، القيء
Loss of appetite or weight gain/loss and diabetes	فقدان الشهية أو زيادة أو خسارة الوزن ومرض السكري
Diarrhoea or constipation	إسهال أو إمساك
Insomnia	الأرق
Confusion	إرتباك
Impaired alertness and motor coordination	ضعف بالتّيقّظ و التناسق الحركي
Worsening of depression or suicidal thinking	تفاقم الاكتئاب والتفكير الانتحاري
Complex sleep behaviours	سلوكيات النوم المعقدة
Sleep paralysis	شلل النوم أو شَلَل اسْتيقاظِيّ
Compromised respiratory function	نقص في وظائف الجهاز التنفسي
Epistaxis	نَزْفٌ أنْفِيّ أو رُعَاف الأنْفِ
Liver or pancreas problems	مشاكل الكبد أو البنكرياس
A serious drop in white blood cells	انخفاض خطير في خلايا الدم البيضاء
A serious drop in the number of platelets	انخفاض خطير في عدد الصفائح الدموية
Aplastic anemia	فَقُرُ الدّمِ اللّاتَنَسُّجِيّ
Liver failure	فشل الكبد
Osteoporosis and fractures	هشاشة العظام والكسور
Reduced sex drive	انخفاض الدافع الجنسي
Erectile dysfunction	خلل بالإنتصاب
Excessive sweating	التعرق المفرط
Arrhythmia	عدم انتظام ضربات القلب
Aspirin-induced asthma	الربو الناجم عن الأسبرين
Serotonin syndrome	متلازمة السيروتونين
Hyponatraemia	نَقْصُ صُوديوم الدّم
Suicidal thoughts	أفكار انتحارية

- ## Neuropsychological Assessment

Many things can affect how our brains function. A person may have an illness or condition that has the potential to affect thinking skills. Some common examples include:
• Epilepsy
• Traumatic Brain injury
• Stroke
• Multiple Sclerosis

يمكن للكثير من الأمور أن تؤثّر على كيفية عمل أدمغتنا. قد يكون لدى الشخص مرض أو حالة من المحتمل أن تؤثر على مهارات التفكير لديه. بعض الأمثلة الشّائعة تتضمّن:

- مرض الصّرع
- إصابة رضحية في الدّماغ
- سكتة دماغية
- التّصلّب اللُّويحي المتعدّد

Or, maybe a patient or their family have noticed a change in thinking skills and they want to get more information about those changes. An assessment can help those involved in patient care to:
• Support a diagnosis.
• Better understand the symptoms.
• Decide what treatment or interventions might be most suited for the patient.
• Track any changes in the patients' thinking skills over time.

أو ربما لاحظ المريض أو أهله تغيّرات في مهاراته الفكرية ويريدون الحصول على معلومات أكثر حول هذه التغيرات. يمكن للتّقييم أن يساعد المشاركين في رعاية المريض على:

- دعم التّشخيص
- فهم أفضل للأعراض
- تحديد العلاج أو التّدخلات الأنسب للمريض
- تتبّع التغيرات في المهارات الفكرية للمريض مع مرور الوقت

The assessment does not require any physical examination or procedures. It is divided into two parts:
1. The Neuropsychologist will ask the patient and family members about medical and personal history, and if the patient has any concerns about their cognition, mood, and function in everyday tasks.
2. Guided by the doctor, the patient will be asked to complete a range of different tasks and puzzles. Each task is designed to use a different part of the brain. The patient may feel like some of the tasks are not very relevant, but they all have a purpose and add to the doctor gaining a complete picture. Most tasks start off easy and gradually get harder. Everyone finds them difficult in the end. They are made that way so that they can capture a wide range of abilities. All the patient needs to do, is to try their best all the way through.

التّقييم لا يتطلّب أي فحوصات أوإجراءات جسديّة. إنها مقسّمة إلى جزأين:
1. سيسألُ الطبيب العصبي النفسي؛ المريض وأهل المريض عن تاريخه الطبي والشخصي، وما إذا كان لدى المريض أي مخاوف بشأن قدراته الفكرية والمزاج وأدائه في المهام اليوميّة.
2. مع توجيه الطبيب، سيُطلب من المريض إكمال مجموعة من المهام والألغاز المختلفة. تم تصميم كل مهمة لاستخدام جزء مختلف من الدّماغ. قد يشعر المريض ان بعض هذه المهام ليست وثيقة الصّلة بالموضوع، ولكن جميعها لها نتائج هامة ستمكّن الطبيب من رسم صورة كاملة لقدرات المريض. تبدأ معظم المهام بسهولة وتصبح تدريجيًّا أكثر صعوبة. الجميع يجد صعوبة في النّهاية. الغاية الرّئيسيّة من هذه المهام هو الحصول على تقييم مبدئي للقدرات. كلّ ما على المريض فعله هو بذل قصارى جهده حتى النهاية.

The assessment usually takes about three hours, but sometimes it can be longer or shorter. The patient is allowed to take a short break if they get tired or need to use the bathroom. Afterwards, the neuropsychologist will analyze all the results and prepare a report for those involved in the patient's care. The report includes:
• A summary of all the background information.
• Details of the assessment results and what they mean.
• Suggestions and recommendations for management and practical support.

يستغرق التّقييم حواليّ ثلاث ساعات، ولكن قد تطول المدّة أو تقصر. يُسمح للمريض بأخذ إستراحة قصيرة إذا أحسّ بالتعب أو إحتاج إلى إستخدام دورة المياه. بعد ذلك، سيقوم الطبيب العصبي النفسي بتحليل جميع النتائج ويُحظّر تقرير لجميع المشتركين في رعاية المريض. سيتضمّن هذا التقرير:
- مُلخّص عن كافّة المعلومات الخلفيّة
- تفاصيل نتائج التقييم وشرح عنها
- إقتراحات وتوصيّات للإدارة والدّعم العمليّ.

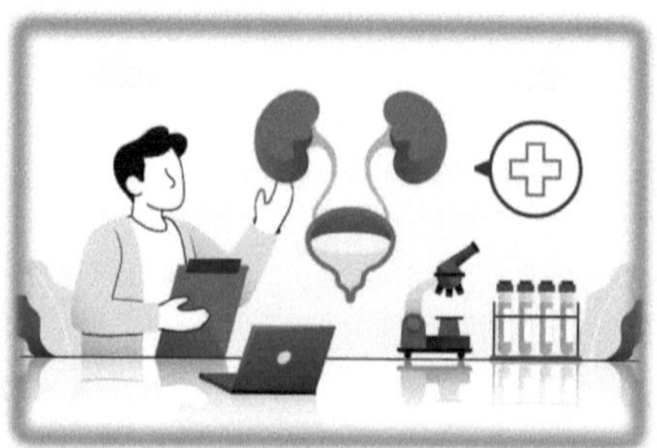

Chapter EIGHT – Urology & Gynecology

Overview

This chapter introduces the reader to common medical terminology of Urology specialty that will include bilingual terminology for the following;

1. Anatomy
2. Common Symptoms
3. Diseases and disorders
4. Common Sexual Diseases / Health Conditions
5. Investigations
6. Surgery / Procedures

We hope you enjoy reading this Chapter, and more chapters awaiting you

URINARY SYSTEM

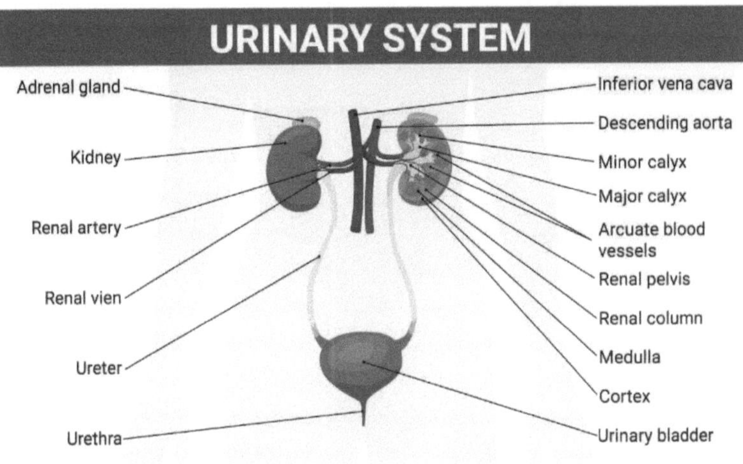

FEMALE REPRODUCTIVE SYSTEM

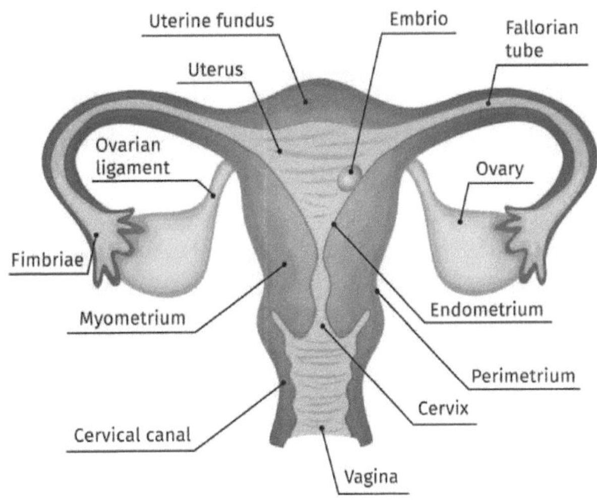

Male reproductive system

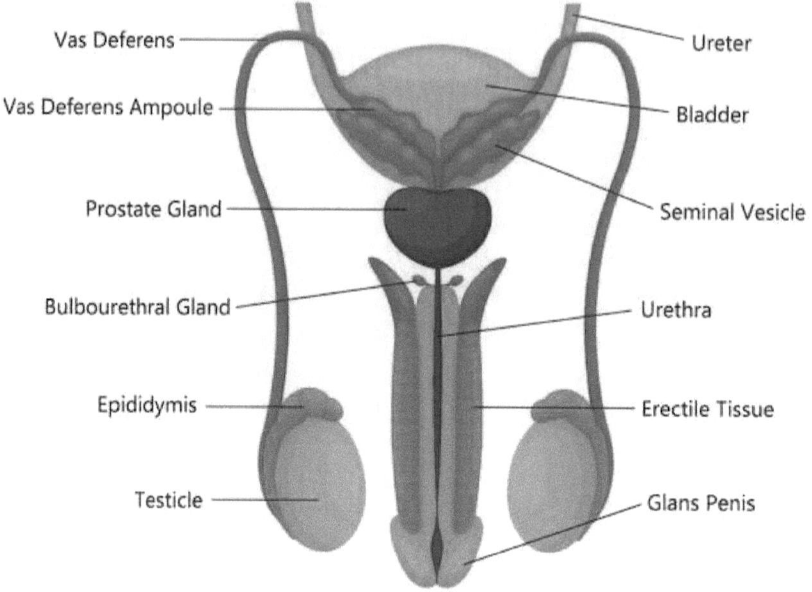

The Common Symptoms

Term	المصطلح
Urinary Tract Symptoms:	أعراض المسالك البولية:
Bed Wetting	التبول الليلي
Erectile Dysfunction	ضعف في الانتصاب
Sexual Dysfunction	ضعف جنسي
Premature Ejaculation	سرعة القذف
Urethral Discharge	إفرازات إحليلية
Hematuria	دم في البول
Incomplete Bladder Emptying	عدم تفريغ كامل للمثانة
Poor flow of Urine	ضعف تدفق البول
Incontinence (difficulty holding urine or leaking)	سلس البول (صعوبة حبس البول أو تسريبه)
Blood in the urine	دم في البول
Pain when you urinate	ألم عند التبول
Changes in urinary pattern	تغيرات في النمط البولي
Frequent need to urinate	كثرة الحاجة للتبول
Inability to urinate	عدم القدرة على التبول
Weak or hesitant urinary stream	ضعف مجرى البول أو تردده
Pain in the lower abdomen	ألم في أسفل البطن
Frequent urinary tract infections	التهابات المسالك البولية المتكررة
Male infertility	عقم الذكور
Male impotence or erectile dysfunction	الضعف الجنسي لدى الذكور أو ضعف الانتصاب
Mass in testicle	ورم في الخصية
Awaking two or more times in the night to urinate	الاستيقاظ مرتين أو أكثر في الليل للتبول
Change in urine color	تغير في لون البول
Cloudy urine	بول غائم
Difficulty emptying bladder or weak urine stream	صعوبة إفراغ المثانة أو ضعف مجرى البول
Difficulty starting urination	صعوبة في بدء التبول
Frequent urination	كثرة التبول
Involuntary loss of urine	فقدان البول اللاإرادي
Pain or burning when urinating	ألم أو حرقة عند التبول
Strong, persistent urge to urinate	إلحاح قوي ومستمر للتبول
Related pain involves	يتضمن الألم ذات الصلة
Itching or burning around genitals, buttocks or inner thighs	حكة أو حرقة حول الأعضاء التناسلية أو الأرداف أو باطن الفخذين
Pain in back or side	ألم في الظهر أو الجانب

Pain in lower abdomen or groin	ألم في أسفل البطن أو الفخذ
Painful ejaculation	القذف المؤلم
Painful sexual intercourse	الجماع المؤلم
Stress	ضغط
Blurred vision	رؤية مشوشة
Bumps, blisters or open sores around genitals	نتوءات أو بثور أو قروح مفتوحة حول الأعضاء التناسلية
Change in vaginal discharge	تغير في الإفرازات المهبلية
Clear discharge from penis	إفرازات واضحة من القضيب
Extreme thirst or hunger	العطش الشديد أو الجوع
Fatigue	تعب
Fever	حمى
Nausea or vomiting	الغثيان أو القيء
Pus-filled discharge from penis	إفرازات مليئة بالصديد من القضيب
Unintended weight loss	فقدان الوزن غير المقصود
Vaginal odor	رائحة من المهبل

The Common Disease/health conditions	
Term	المصطلح
Urinary tract infection	التهاب المسالك البولية
Undescended Testicle	الخصية المعلقة
Kidney Stone	حصى الكلى
Benign prostatic hyperplasia	تضخم البروستاتا الحميد
Urethritis	التهاب الإحليل
Testicular pain	ألم خصوي
Hypercalcemia	فرط كالسيوم الدم
Cystitis	التهاب المثانة
Nephrocalcinosis	تكلس الكلى
Urinary incontinence	السلس البولي
Recurrent Urinary Tract Infection - UTI	التهاب المسالك البولية المتكررة
Inborn anomalies of the genitourinary tract	العيوب الخلقية في المسالك البولية
Chronic prostatitis (Chronic pelvic pain syndrome - SPPS)	التهاب البروستاتا المزمن- متلازمة الام الحوض المزمنة
The over active bladder	المثانة مفرطة النشاط
Hematuria	البيلة الدموية
Nephrotic syndrome in adults	المتلازمة الكلائية لدى البالغين
Renal Tubular Acidosis	حماضّ كلوئ نبيبي
Cystinuria	بيلة سيستينية
The Nephrotic syndrome	المتلازمة الكلائية
Cystocele	قيلة مثانية
Urolithiasis	تحصٍ بولي
Polycystic kidney disease	مرض الكلية متعددة الكيسات
Uremic frost	الصقيع اليوريمي
IgA nephropathy	اعتلال الكلى بالغلوبيين المناعي أ
Cystinosis	الداء السيستيني
Nephroblastoma	الورم الأرومي الكلوي
Azothemia	الازوتيمية
Pyelonephritis	التهاب الحويضة والكلية
Congenital hydronephrosis	موه الكلية الخلقي
Bladder cancer	سرطان المثانة
Nocturia	التبول الليلي
Chronic Renal Failure	الفشل الكلوي
Renal Colic	المغص الكلوي
Benign Prostate Enlargement	البروستاتا

Incontinence	سلس البول
Adrenal Gland Cancers	سرطان الغدة الكظرية
Adrenal Mass	كتلة الغدة الكظرية
Ambiguous (Uncertain) Genitalia	الأعضاء التناسلية المبهمة (غير مؤكدة)
Benign Prostatic Hyperplasia (BPH)	تضخم البروستاتا الحميد(BPH)
Benign (Not Cancerous) Urethral Lesions	آفات مجرى البول الحميدة (غير السرطانية)
Benign (Not Cancerous) Uretheral Lesions Boys	آفات مجرى البول الحميدة (غير السرطانية)
Benign (Not Cancerous) Uretheral Lesions Girls	آفات مجرى البول الحميدة (غير السرطانية)
Bladder Augmentation (Enlargement)	تكبير المثانة (تكبير)
Bladder Diverticulum	رتج المثانة
Bladder Dysfunction and Urine Control in Children	ضعف المثانة والسيطرة على البول عند الاطفال
Bladder Exstrophy	انقلاب المثانة للخارج
Bladder Fistula	ناسور المثانة
Bladder Prolapse (Cystocele)	تدلي المثانة (القيلة المثانية)
Bladder Trauma	إصابات المثانة
Circumcision	الختان
Cloacal Exstrophy	كلوكال إكستروفي
Conn's Syndrome	متلازمة كون
Cryptorchidism	الخصية الخفية
Cushing's Syndrome	متلازمة كوشينغ
Ectopic Kidney	الكلى خارج الرحم
Ectopic Ureter	الحالب خارج الرحم
Epididymitis and Orchitis	التهاب البربخ والتهاب الخصية
Epispadias (A congenital malformation where the urethra opens into the penis, or the glans.)	مبال فوقاني (تشوه خلقي حيث يفتح الإحليل في ظهر القضيب، أو في الحشفة.)
Erectile Dysfunction (ED)	ضعف الانتصاب(ED)
Extrinsic Obstruction of the Ureter	انسداد خارجي للحالب
Hematuria	بيلة دموية
Horseshoe Kidney (Renal Fusion)	كلية حدوة الحصان (الانصهار الكلوي)
Hydroceles and Inguinal Hernia	القيلة المائية والفتق الأربي
Hypospadias	إحليل تحتي
Immunotherapy and Bladder Cancer	العلاج المناعي وسرطان المثانة
Interstitial Cystitis	التهاب المثانة الخلالي

Kidney Cancer	سرطان الكلى
Kidney Cancer in Children	سرطان الكلى عند الأطفال
Kidney (Renal) Abscess	خراج كلوي
Kidney (Renal) Dysplasia and Cystic Disease	خلل التنسج الكلوي والمرض الكيسي
Kidney (Renal) Failure	الفشل الكلوي
Kidney (Renal) Infection - Pyelonephritis	عدوى الكلى - التهاب الحويضة والكلية
Kidney (Renal) Trauma	رضوض الكلى (كلوية)
Kidney Stones	حصوات الكلى
Kidney Transplant	زراعة الكلى
Low Testosterone	انخفاض هرمون التستوستيرون
Male Infertility	العقم عند الرجال
Meatal Stenosis	تَضيُّق إحليلي (مجرى البول)
Megaureter	توسع الحالب
Muscle Invasive Bladder Cancer	سرطان المثانة الغازي للعضلات
Neonatal Testicular Torsion	التواء الخصية الوليدي
Neurogenic Bladder	المثانة العصبية
Nocturia	التبول الليلي
Nocturnal Enuresis (Bedwetting)	سلس البول الليلي (التبول اللاإرادي)
Non-muscle Invasive Bladder Cancer	سرطان المثانة غير الغازي للعضلات
Overactive Bladder (OAB)	فرط نشاط المثانة(OAB)
Paruresis (Urinating in Public)	التبول في الأماكن العامة (Paruresis)
Pelvic Floor Muscles	عضلات قاع الحوض
Penile Augmentation	تكبير القضيب
Penile Cancer	سرطان القضيب
Penile Trauma	إصابة القضيب
Peyronie's Disease	مرض بيروني
Pheochromocytoma (Adrenal Medulla Tumor)	ورم القواتم (ورم النخاع الكظري)
Premature Ejaculation	سرعة القذف
Priapism	القساح
Prostate Cancer – Advanced	سرطان البروستاتا – متقدم
Prostate Cancer – Early-Stage	سرطان البروستاتا - مرحلة مبكرة
Prostatitis (Infection of the Prostate)	التهاب البروستاتا (التهاب البروستاتا)
Renal Mass and Localized Renal Tumors	الكتلة الكلوية والأورام الكلوية الموضعية
Renovascular Disease	أمراض الأوعية الدموية الكلوية
Retrograde Urethrogram	رجوع مجرى البول

Rhabdomyosarcoma	الساركوما العضلية المخططة
Sexually Transmitted Infections	الأمراض التي تنتقل عن طريق الاتصال الجنسي
Spermatoceles	القيلة المنوية
Sperm Retrieval	استرجاع الحيوانات المنوية
Stress Urinary Incontinence (SUI)	سلس البول الإجهادي(SUI)
Testicular Cancer	سرطان الخصية
Testicular Cancer in Children	سرطان الخصية عند الأطفال
Testicular Torsion	التواء الخصية
Testicular Trauma	صدمة الخصية
Upper Urinary Tract Cancer	سرطان المسالك البولية العلوية
Urachal Abnormalities	تشوهات أوراشال
Ureterocele	قيلة حالبية
Ureteropelvic Junction (UPJ) Obstruction	انسداد مفرق الحالب(UPJ)
Urethral Cancer	سرطان الإحليل
Urethral Diverticulum	رتج مجرى البول
Urethral Stricture Disease	مرض تضيق مجرى البول
Urethral Trauma	صدمة مجرى البول
Urinary Incontinence	سلس البول
Urinary Diversion	تحويل مجرى البول
Urinary Tract Infections in Adults	التهابات المسالك البولية عند البالغين
Urinary Tract Infections in Children	التهابات المسالك البولية عند الأطفال
Urotrauma	صدمات البول
Vaginal Abnormalities: Cloacal Abnormalities	تشوهات المهبل: شذوذ في فتحة الشرج
Vaginal Abnormalities: Congenital Vaginal Obstruction	تشوهات المهبل: انسداد مهبلي خلقي
Vaginal Abnormalities: Fusion and Duplication	تشوهات المهبل: اندماج وازدواج
Vaginal Abnormalities: Urogenital Sinus	تشوهات المهبل: الجيوب البولية التناسلية
Vaginal Abnormalities: Vaginal Agenesis	تشوهات المهبل: عدم تخلق المهبل
Varicoceles	دوالي الخصية
Vasectomy	قطع القناة الدافقة
Vasectomy Reversal	عكس قطع القناة الدافقة
Vesicoureteral Reflux (VUR)	الجزر المثاني الحالبي(VUR)
Yeast Infections	عدوى الخميرة
Benign Prostatic Hyperplasia	تضخم البروستاتا الحميد
Hydronephrosis	تضخم الكلى

- The Common Sexual Diseases / Health Conditions

The Common Disease/health conditions	
Term	المصطلح
Bacterial Vaginosis	التهاب المهبل البكتيري
BV is a common, treatable, vaginal condition which can increase your chance of getting an STD.	التهاب المهبل البكتيري هو حالة مهبلية شائعة يمكن علاجها ويمكن أن تزيد من فرصتك في الإصابة بالأمراض المنقولة بالاتصال الجنسي.
Chlamydia	الكلاميديا
Chlamydia is a common, but treatable, STD. If left untreated, chlamydia can make it difficult for a woman to get pregnant.	الكلاميديا من الأمراض المنقولة بالاتصال الجنسي الشائعة ولكن يمكن علاجها. إذا تُركت دون علاج ، يمكن أن تجعل الكلاميديا من الصعب على المرأة الحمل.
Gonorrhea	السيلان
Gonorrhea is a common STD that can be treated with the right medication. If left untreated, gonorrhea can cause very serious health problems.	السيلان هو مرض منتشر يمكن علاجه بالأدوية المناسبة. إذا تركت دون علاج ، يمكن أن يسبب مرض السيلان مشاكل صحية خطيرة للغاية.
Hepatitis	التهاب الكبد
Viral hepatitis is the leading cause of liver cancer and the most common reason for liver transplants.	التهاب الكبد الفيروسي هو السبب الرئيسي لسرطان الكبد والسبب الأكثر شيوعًا لعمليات زرع الكبد.
Herpes	الهربس
Genital herpes is a common STD, but most people with the infection do not know they have it. While there is no cure, there are medicines available that can prevent or shorten outbreaks. These medicines also can make it less likely to pass the infection on.	الهربس التناسلي من الأمراض التي تنتقل عن طريق الاتصال الجنسي ، ولكن معظم المصابين بالعدوى لا يعرفون أنهم مصابون بها. على الرغم من عدم وجود علاج ، إلا أن هناك أدوية يمكن أن تمنع أو تقلل من تفشي المرض. يمكن لهذه الأدوية أيضًا أن تقلل من احتمالية نقل العدوى.
HIV/AIDS & STDs	فيروس نقص المناعة البشرية / الإيدز والأمراض المنقولة جنسيا
Human Papillomavirus (HPV) Infection	عدوى فيروس الورم الحليمي البشري
HPV is the most common STI in the United States, but most people with the infection have no symptoms. HPV can cause some health effects that are preventable with vaccines.	فيروس الورم الحليمي البشري هو أكثر أنواع العدوى المنقولة جنسيًا شيوعًا في الولايات المتحدة ، ولكن معظم المصابين بالعدوى لا تظهر عليهم أعراض. يمكن أن يسبب فيروس الورم الحليمي البشري بعض الآثار الصحية التي يمكن الوقاية منها باللقاحات.
Mycoplasma genitalium (Mgen)	Mycoplamsa genitalium ، أو Mgen
Mycoplamsa genitalium, or Mgen is an STD that can be treated with antibiotics. People receiving treatment for Mgen should take all of the medication as prescribed.	هو مرض منقول جنسياً يمكن علاجه بالمضادات الحيوية. يجب على الأشخاص الذين يتلقون علاج Mgen أن يأخذوا جميع الأدوية على النحو الموصوف.
Pelvic Inflammatory Disease (PID)	مرض التهاب الحوض (PID)
PID can lead to serious consequences including infertility.	يمكن أن يؤدي مرض التهاب الحوض إلى عواقب وخيمة بما في ذلك العقم.
STDs & Infertility	الأمراض المنقولة بالاتصال الجنسي والعقم
Chlamydia and gonorrhea can cause PID and infertility, but both are preventable.	يمكن أن تسبب الكلاميديا والسيلان مرض التهاب الحوض والعقم ، ولكن يمكن الوقاية من كليهما.
Syphilis	مرض الزهري

Syphilis can have very serious problems when left untreated. It is simple to cure with the right treatment.	يمكن أن يعاني مرض الزهري من مشاكل خطيرة للغاية عند تركه دون علاج. من السهل علاجه بالعلاج الصحيح.
Trichomoniasis Most people who have trichomoniasis do not have any symptoms.	داء المشعرات لا تظهر أي أعراض على معظم المصابين بداء المشعرات.
Other STDs	**الأمراض المنقولة بالاتصال الجنسي الأخرى**
Chancroid, scabies	Chancroid والجرب
- Erectile dysfunction	ضعف الانتصاب -
- Postcoital bleeding	نزيف ما بعد ممارسة الجنس -
- Anal sexually transmitted diseases	الأمراض المنقولة بالجنس الشرجي -
- Lymphogranuloma venereum	الورم الحبيبي اللمفي المنقول جنسيا -
- Condyloma lata	ورمٌ لقميٌّ مسطح -
- Female Sexual Dysfunction	الاضطراب الجنسي لدى النساء Female -
- Gynecomastia	التثدي عند الرجال -
- Hypogonadism	قصور الغدد التناسلية -
- Dyspareunia	عسر الجماع -
- Precocious puberty	البلوغ المبكر -
- Menopause	انقطاع الدورة الشهرية -
- Contraception	وسائل منع الحمل -
- Sexually transmitted disease	الأمراض المنقولة جنسيًا –
- Congenital syphilis	الزهري الخلقي -
- Congenital anomalies - Mulerian system	عيوب خلقية في الجهاز التناسلي -
- Penile curvature	انحناء القضيب -
- Ureoplasma urealyticum	الميورة الحالة لليوريا -
- Premature Ejaculation	سرعة القذف -
- Impotence - erectile dysfunction	الاضطرابات الجنسية - -
- Paraphilia	التحرش الجنسي -
- Pedophilia	عشق الأطفال -
- Vaginal Yeast Infection	الفطريات المهبلية -

- Investigations

Diagnostic Service	المصطلح
Radiology	
X-ray	الأشعة السينية
CT Scan	الاشعة المقطعية
Magnetic Resonance Imaging (MRI)	التصوير بالرنين المغناطيسي (مري)
Ultrasound Imaging	التصوير بالموجات فوق الصوتية
Ultrasonography and Doppler Sonography (for evaluation of erectile problems)	
Bladder Scan (Radionuclide Cystogram)	مسح المثانة (مخطط النويدات المشعة)
Kidney (Renal) Nuclear Medicine Scan	مسح الكلى (الكلى) الطب النووي
Urologic Radiology	أشعة المسالك البولية
Angiography	تصوير الأوعية
Laboratory	
Complete Blood Count (CBC)	تعداد الدم الكامل (CBC)
Antegrade Pyelography	تَصْويرُ الحُوَيضَةِ بالحَقُن المُباشِر
Biopsy	خزعة
Urinalysis	تحليل البول
Urine Culture Sample	عينة مزرعة البول
Urine Cystology	كيس البول
Urodynamics	ديناميكا البول
Uroflowmetry	قياس جريان البول
Voiding Cystourethrogram	تفريغ المثانة والإحليل
Cystometry	قياس المثانة
Cystoscopy	تنظير المثانة
Intravenous Pyelogram (IVP)	تصوير الحويضة في الوريد (IVP)
Retrograde Pyelography	رجوع الحويضة
Testicular Self-Exam	الفحص الذاتي للخصيتين

- Surgery / Procedures

Surgery / Procedures	
Term	المصطلح
Endoscopic surgeries- TURP, PCNL, Laser Surgery for stones, Cystoscopy.	جراحات المناظير- TURP، PCNL ، جراحة الحصوات بالليزر ، تنظير المثانة.
ESWL (Shock wave treatment for stone diseases)	ESWL (علاج الموجات الصدمية لأمراض الحصيات)
Retrograde Intrarenal Surgery (RIRS) For Difficult Renal Stones / Renal Problems	الجراحة الارتجاعية داخل الكلى (RIRS) لحصوات الكلى الصعبة / مشاكل الكلى
Microsurgical Varicocelectomy.	استئصال القيلة الدوالية بالجراحة المجهرية.
Hydrocelectomy	استئصال القيلة المائية
Urology Laparoscopic Procedures	إجراءات جراحة المسالك البولية بالمنظار
Kidney, ureteral and bladder stone treatment	علاج حصوات الكلى والحالب والمثانة
Incontinence treatment	علاج سلس البول
Urologic Tumors and Oncology	أورام المسالك البولية والأورام
Targeted ultrasound-guided biopsy of the prostate	خزعة البروستاتا الموجهة بالموجات فوق الصوتية
Endourology for stone disease (kidney, ureter, and bladder)	طب الجهاز البولي لأمراض الحصيات (الكلى والحالب والمثانة)
Laser treatment of stones	علاج الحصوات بالليزر
Endoscopic diagnostics of prostate, bladder, ureter, and kidney as well as urethral diseases with latest world-class technologies (small flexible instruments, etc.)	التشخيصات التنظيرية للبروستاتا والمثانة والحالب والكلى وكذلك أمراض الإحليل بأحدث التقنيات العالمية (أدوات مرنة صغيرة ، إلخ)
Botox injection for overactive bladder	حقن البوتوكس لفرط نشاط المثانة
Prostate surgery including minimal invasive techniques	جراحة البروستاتا بما في ذلك تقنيات الحد الأدنى من التدخل الجراحي
Surgery for urethral stricture	جراحة تضيق مجرى البول
Surgery of bladder tumor	جراحة ورم المثانة
Varicocele treatment (radiological embolization and micro-surgical ligation)	علاج دوالي الخصية (الانصمام الشعاعي والربط الجراحي الدقيق)
Vasectomy and vasectomy reversal	قطع القناة الدافقة وعكس قطع القناة المنوية
Scrotal surgery (Orchidectomy Hydrocelectomy, spermatocele excision etc.)	جراحة كيس الصفن (استئصال القيلة المائية ، استئصال القيلة المنوية ، إلخ)
Surgical sperm retrieval	سحب الحيوانات المنوية جراحيًا
Insertion of penile implant for end stage erectile dysfunction	إدخال الدعامة القضيبية في المرحلة النهائية من ضعف الانتصاب

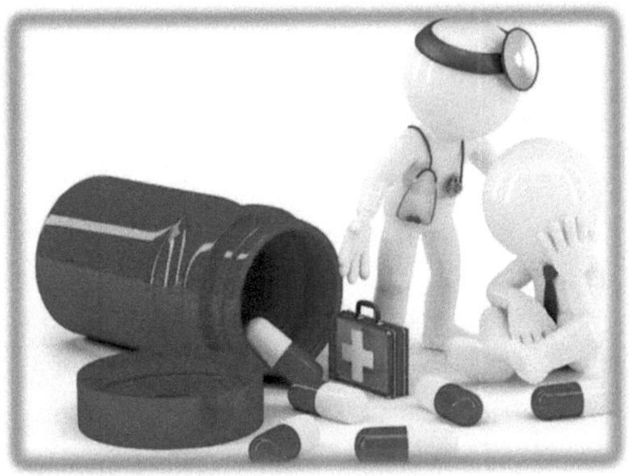 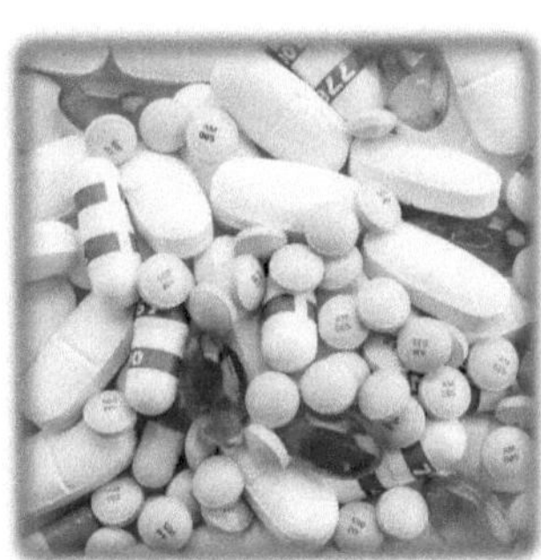

Chapter NINE- Medication and Pain Descriptor

Overview

This chapter introduces the reader to common medical terminology of Medication and Pain Descriptor that will include bilingual terminology for the following;

6. General Drug Categories
7. Antihypertensives
8. Anti-anginal Agents
9. Allergy, Cough and Cold Medications
10. Medications used in Peptic Ulcer Disease
11. Other Gastrointestinal Medications
12. Medications to treat Ear Problems
13. Medications to treat Skin Problems
14. Pain Descriptor
15. Route of Medications Administration

We hope you enjoy reading this Chapter, and more chapters awaiting you

- **General Drug Categories**

Term	Synonym		Term	Synonym	
Analgesics	Pain killer	مسكن ألم	Cold Cures		علاجات البرد
Antacids		مضادات الحموضة	Corticosteroids		الستيرويدات القشرية
Antianxiety Drugs		الأدوية المضادة للقلق	Cough Suppressants		مثبطات السعال
Antiarrhythmics		مضاد لاضطراب النظم	Cytotoxics		السموم الخلوية
Antibacterials		مضادات الجراثيم	Decongestants		مزيلات الاحتقان
Antibiotics		مضادات حيوية	Diuretics		مدرات البول
Anticoagulants and Thrombolytics		مضادات التخثر ومزيلات التخثر	Expectorant	apophlegmatic	طارد للبلغم
Anticonvulsants		مضادات الاختلاج (التشنج)	Hormones		الهرمونات
Antidepressants		مضادات الاكتئاب	Hypoglycemics (Oral)		مخفض للسكر (عن طريق الفم)
Antidiarrheals		مضادات الإسهال	Immunosuppressives		مثبطات المناعة
Antiemetics		مضادات القيء	Laxatives		المسهلات
Antifungals		مضادات الفطريات	Muscle Relaxants		مرخيات العضلات
Antihistamines		مضادات الهيستامين (للحساسية)	Sedatives	calmative	المهدئات, منوم
Antihypertensives		خافضات ضغط الدم	Sex Hormones (Female)		هرمونات الجنس (أنثى)
Anti-Inflammatories		مضادات الالتهاب	Sex Hormones (Male)		هرمونات الجنس (ذكر)
Antineoplastics		مضادات الأورام	Sleeping Drugs		أدوية النوم
Antipsychotics		مضادات الذهان	Tranquilizer		مهدئ للأعصاب
Antipyretics		خافضات الحرارة			
Antivirals		مضادات الفيروسات			
Barbiturates		الباربيتورات			
Beta-Blockers		حاصرات بيتا			
Bronchodilators		موسعات الشعب الهوائية			

- **Antihypertensives**

Antihypertensives			
خافضات ضغط الدم			
Type of Drug		What does it do?	Examples
Diuretics	مدرات البول	Help the body to make more urine by making the kidneys give up more salts and water. Diuretics are used to treat swelling (edema), high blood pressure (hypertension) or congestive heart failure.	Amiloride Dyazide Furosemide Hydrochlorothiazide Maxide Spironolactone Triamterene
Vasodilators	موسعات الأوعية	Relax the arterial walls, making it easier for the blood to flow through the blood vessels and lowering high blood pressure.	Hydralazine Minoxidil
Beta-blockers	حاصرات (معوقات) بيتا	Block certain cells in the heart called "beta receptors": this decreases the activity of the heart and lowers blood pressure.	Atenolol Labetalol Metoprolol Nadolol Pindolol Propranolol
Angiotensin-converting enzyme inhibitors (ACE inhibitors)	مثبطات الإنزيم المحول للأنجيوتنسين	If angiotensin I converts to angiotensin II, blood pressure increases. ACE inhibitors block this conversion, and so lower blood pressure.	Benazepril Captopril Enalapril Lisinopril
Other antihypertensives	خافضات ضغط الدم أخرى		Clonidine Guanabez Guanfacine Prazosin Reserpine

- **Anti-anginal Agents**

<table>
<tr><td colspan="4" align="center">Anti-anginal Agents</td></tr>
<tr><td colspan="4" align="center">مضاد الذبحة الصدرية</td></tr>
<tr><td>Type of Drug</td><td></td><td>What does it do?</td><td>Examples</td></tr>
<tr><td>Nitrites</td><td>النتريت</td><td>The heart's need for oxygen and improves the flow ofblood to the heart tissues.</td><td>• Isosorbide Nitroglyce rine</td></tr>
<tr><td>Calcium channel blockers</td><td>مثبط قناة الكالسيوم</td><td>Prevent and reverse heart spasm by stopping the flow of calcium into the muscles of the heart. This improves the blood flow, which increases the amount of oxygen reaching the heart and reverses angina pectoris.</td><td>• Diltiazem Nifedipine Verapamil</td></tr>
<tr><td>Beta-blockers</td><td>حاصرات (معوقات) بيتا</td><td>Control angina by reducing the heart's need for oxygen.</td><td>• Propranol ol</td></tr>
<tr><td>Peripheral vasodilators</td><td>موسعات الأوعية المحيطية</td><td>Relax the blood vessels, making it easier for the blood to flow and increasing the amount of blood that can reach the heart.</td><td></td></tr>
</table>

Allergy, Cough and Cold Medications

أدوية الحساسية، السعال، والبرد

Type of Drug		What does it do?	Examples
Antihistamines	مضادات الهيستامين (للحساسية)	Relieve mild symptoms such as allergic rhinitis sneezing, runny nose, hay fever, watery eyes, and pruritus.	Astemazole (Hismanal) Brompheniramine (Dimetane) Ceterizine (Zyrtec) Chlorpheniramine (Chlortrimeton) Dimetapp Diphenhydramine (Benadryl) Loratidine (Claritin) Terfenadine (Seldane)
Nasal decongestants	مزيلات احتقان الأنف	Decrease nasal congestion due to hay fever, allergic rhinitis, sinusitis, and the common cold.	Ephedrine Naphazoline Oxymetazoline Phenylephrine Phenylpropanolamine Pseudophedrine (Sudafed)
Intra-nasal steroids	استيرويد أنفي	Exert local anti-inflammatory effects to relieve symptoms of rhinitis.	Beclomethasone (Beconase, Vancenase) Flunisolide (Nasalide) Triamcinolone (Nasacort)
Narcotic anti-tussive	مضادات السعال (الكحة) المخدرة	Decrease Cough.	Codeine
Non-narcotic Anti-tussives	مضادات السعال (الكحة) الغير مخدرة	Control cough spasms by depressing the coug center in the brain.	Dextromethorphan (Delsym) Diphenhydramine (Benadryl)Benzonatate (Tessalon)
Expectorants Or apophlegmatic	طارد للبلغم	Help the patient cough up mucous from the lungs; used for cough,	Guaifenesin Iodinited glycerol (Organidin)Potassium Iodide Tepin Hydrate

Medications used in Peptic Ulcer Disease

أدوية القرحة الهضمية

Type of Drug		What does it do?	Examples
Antacids	مضاد للحموضة	Neutralize stomach acid. By lessening the acid in the stomach, antacids help reduce pain from stomach ulcers.	Malox Mylant a Tums
H2 antagonists (Histamine 2 blockers)	مضادات الهيستامين النوع الثاني (للحساسية)	Block the production of histamine at the H_2 receptors in the digestive system, which helps to decrease the amount of acid in the stomach.	Cimetidine (Tagamet) Famotidine (Pepcid) Nizatidine (Axid) Ranitidine (Zantac)
Proton pump Inhibitors	مثبطات مضخة البروتون	Block acid production by inhibiting certain enzymes in the stomach cells.	Lansoprazole (Prevacid) Omeprazole (Prilosec)
Sucralfate		Sticks to the surface of the ulcer, forming a protective barrier against stomach acid.	Sucralfate
Gastro-intestinal anticholinergics	مضادات الكولين المَعِدِي المِعوي	Are used to relieve duodenal ulcer pain. These are used together with other medications to treat ulcers.	Atropine Belladonna products Propantheline
Antibiotics	مضادات حيوية	Are used in combination with other medicines to treat H. Pyloris, a bacteria that causes ulcers.	Amoxicillin Clarithromycin (Biaxin) Metronidazole (Flagyl) Tetracycline
Prostaglandins	بروستاغلاندين أو البروستاديل	Lessens the production of stomach acids and guard the stomach lining from damage caused by NSAIDS (nonsteroidal anti-inflammatory drugs) and aspitin.	Misoprostol (Cytotec)

Other Gastrointestinal Medications			
	أدوية أخرى - الجهاز الهضمي		
Type of Drug		**What does it do?**	**Examples**
Laxatives	الملينات المسهلات	Help the patient have bowl movements more easily.	**Bisacodyl (Ducolax) Docusate (Colace) Fleet enema Glycerin suppository Lactulose Milk of magnesiaMineral oil Psyllium (Metamucil. Correctol)Senna (Senokot)**
Antidiarrheals	مضادات الاسهال	Treat and control diarrhea.	**Bismuth subsalicylate (Pepto-Bismol) Diphenoxylate HCI with Atropine sulfate (Lomotil) Kapectolin with Paregoric Lactobacillius (Lactinex) Lopearmide (Imodium)**
Medication sused for ulcerative Colitis	التهاب القولون التقرحي	Treat ulcerative colitis, which is a condition in whichthe colon becomes inflamed and ulcerated.	Mesalamine (Rowasa) Olsalazine (Dipentum)

- **Medications to treat Ear Problems**

<table>
<tr><td colspan="4" align="center">Medications to treat Ear Problems</td></tr>
<tr><td colspan="4" align="center">أدوية لعلاج مشاكل الأذن</td></tr>
<tr><td>Type of Drug</td><td></td><td align="center">What does it do?</td><td align="center">Examples</td></tr>
<tr><td>Steroid and antibiotic combinations</td><td>تركيبات الستيرويد والمضادات الحيوية</td><td>Are used to treat superficial bacterial infections of the external ear canal.</td><td>Cortisporin Otic
Antibiotic ear solution</td></tr>
<tr><td>Medication for ear pain</td><td>مسكنات ألم الأذن</td><td>Are used to treat ear pain.</td><td>VoSol Otic
VoSol HC
OticAuralgan
Allergen Ear Drops
Acetic Acid Otic</td></tr>
<tr><td>Carbamide</td><td>كرباميد</td><td>Is used to remove ear wax.</td><td>Debrox Drops
Carbamide Ear Drops
Auro Ear Drops</td></tr>
</table>

Medications to treat Skin Problems

أدوية لعلاج مشاكل الجلد

Type of Drug		What does it do?	Examples
Acne products	حب الشباب (العُد)	Are used for topicaltreatment of acne.	Malox Mylanta Tums Benzamycin Benzoyl Peroxide Clindamycin (Cleocin T) Erythromycin (A/T/S) Isotretinoin (Acutane) Metronidazole (Metrogel) Retin-A Sulfacete-R Lotion Tetracycline (Topicycline)
Antiseborrheic products	مضاد للزهم (القشرة أو المثّ)	Are used to treat dandruff and seborrheic dermatitis ofthe scalp.	Betadine Shampoo DHS Tar Shampoo Sebutone Shampoo Selenium sulfide lotion Sulfacetamide lotion (Sebizon)
Topical antihistamines	مضادات الهيستامين الموضعية	Are used for temporally relieve of itching due to minor skin disorders like hives, sunburn, or nonpoisonous insect bite.	Benadryl cream/spray Calamycin Sting Relief
Topical Antiviral Agents	مضادات الفيروسية الموضعية	Are used to treat viral infections of the skin.	Acyclovir Ointment (Zovirax)
Topical Antibiotics	المضادات الحيوية الموضعية	Are used to treat bacterialinfections of the skin.	Bacitracin ointment Erythomycin ointment Gentamicin ointment Mupirocin ointment Neomycin ointment/cream Neosporin ointment/cream Triple anibiotic ointment.
Topical Antifungal Agents	مضادات الفطريات الموضعية	Are used to treat fungalinfections of the skin.	Amphoerecing B cream (Fungizone)Cilopirox cream (Loprox) Clotrimazole cream (Lotrimin) Econazole Cream (Spectazone) Ketoconazole (Nizoral) Miconazole (Monistat-Derm)

	Naftifine cream (Naftin)
	Nystatin cream (Mycostatin)
	Oxiconazole cream (Oxistat)
	Tolnaftate cream (Tinactin)

- ## Pain Descriptors

#	Pain		#	Pain	
	Acute pain	ألم حاد		Pins and Needles	دبابيس وابر
	Aching pain	ألم مؤلم		Pounding	ألم قاصف
	Annoying pain	ألم مزعج		Radiating pain	ألم منتشر
	Bothersome pain	ألم شاق		Sharp pain	ألم حاد
	Burning pain	ألم حارق		Shifting pain	ألم متنقل
	Chronic pain	ألم مزمن		Shooting pain	ألم ناخر
	Comes and goes	ألم في بعض الأحيان (يظهر ويختفي)		Sickening pain	إحساس بالإعياء
	Constant pain	ألم مستمر		Soreness	حرقان
	Cramps	تشنجات وتقلصات		Spasm	تشنج
	Crushing pain	ألم ساحق		Stabbing pain	ألم قاطع مقل السكين
	Cutting pain	ألم قاطع		Stinging pain	ألم لاذع
	Dull pain	ألم غير محدد الوصف		Tenderness	ألم عند اللمس
	Gnawing pain	ألم أكالاً (الإحساس بتآكل)		Throbbing pain	ألم نابض
	Intermittent pain	ألم متقطع		Tingling	ألم مثل الوخز
	Nauseating pain	ألم مسبب للغثيان واللوعة			
	Numbing pain	ألم به تخدر وتنميل			
	Piercing pain	ألم ثاقب			

PAIN MEASUREMENT SCALE

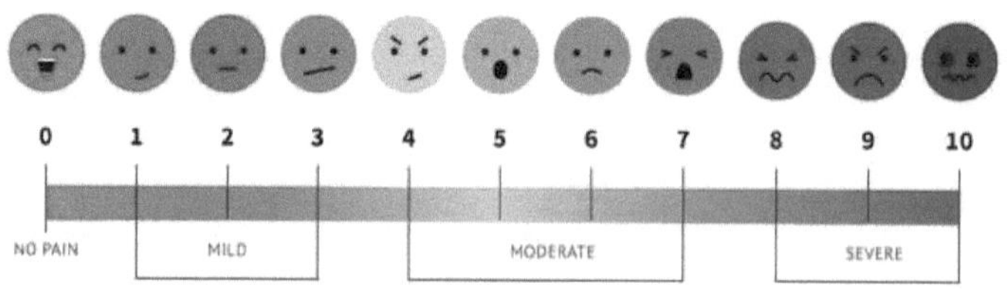

- **Routes of medication administration**

Method		Details
Buccal	وَجنيّ, شدقيّا	held inside the cheek
Enteral	معوي	delivered directly into the stomach or intestine (with a G-tube or J-tube)
Inhalable	مستنشق	breathed in through a tube or mask
Infused	محقونة في الوريد	injected into a vein with an IV line and slowly dripped in over time
Intramuscular (IM injection)	الحقن في العضل	injected into muscle with a syringe
Intrathecal	الحيّز حولَ الحبل الشوكي (داخل القراب)	injected into your spine
Intravenous (IV injection)	الحقن في الوريد	injected into a vein or into an IV line
Nasal	عن طريق الأنف	given into the nose by spray or pump
Ophthalmic	عن طريق العين	given into the eye by drops, gel, or ointment
Oral	عن طريق الفم	swallowed by mouth as a tablet, capsule, lozenge, or liquid
Otic	عن طريق الأذن	given by drops into the ear
Rectal	عن طريق المستقيم	inserted into the rectum
Subcutaneous	تحت الجلد	injected just under the skin
Sublingual	تحت اللسان	held under the tongue
Topical	سطحي	applied to the skin
Transdermal	عبر الجلد	given through a patch placed on the skin

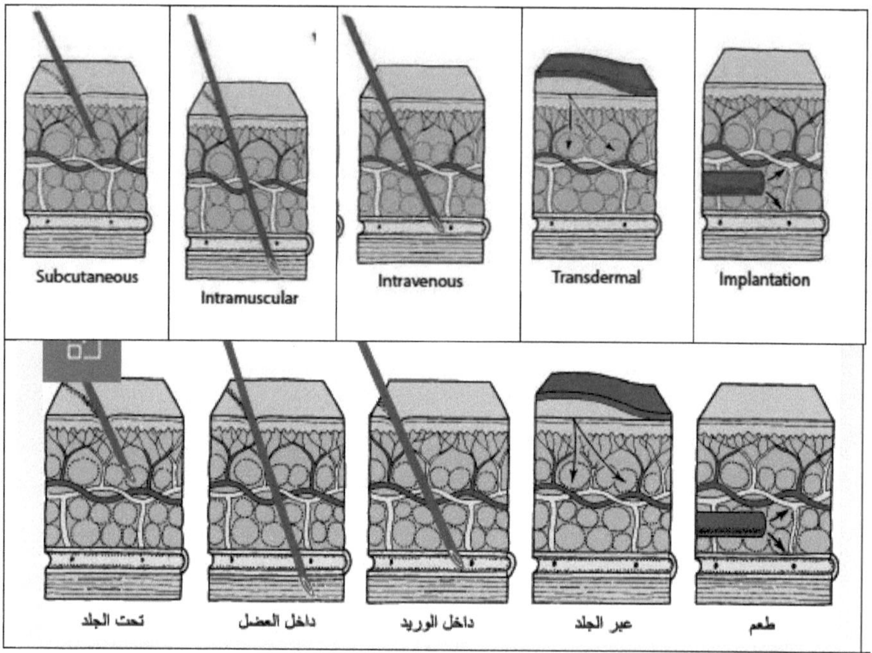

- **Types of injections**

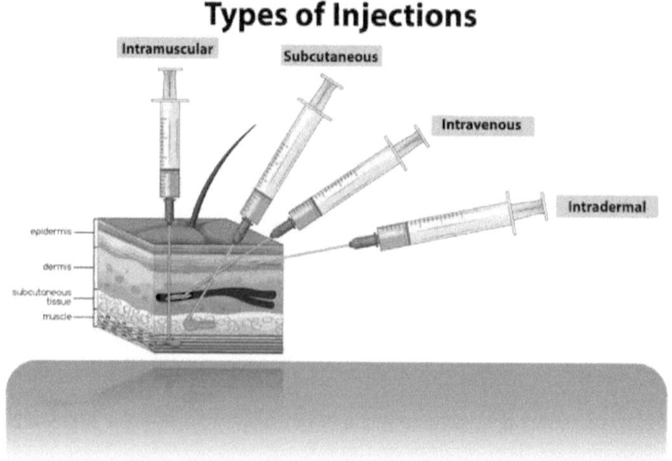

Tests, Investigations & Examinations

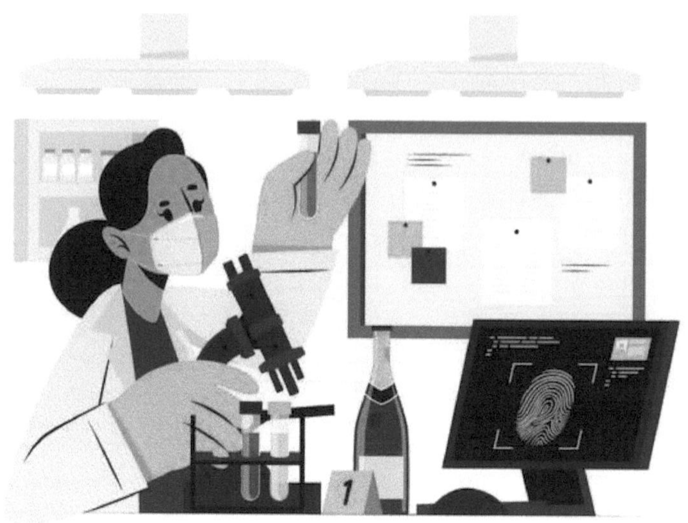

Chapter TEN - Tests, Investigations & Examinations

Overview

This chapter introduces the reader to common medical terminology of All Tests and Investigations that will include bilingual terminology for the following;

- Laboratory
- Radiology
- Physical examinations
- Vitamins and Minerals

We hope you enjoy reading this Chapter, and more chapters awaiting you

- ## TESTS AND INVESTIGATIONS ALPHABETICAL (A…..Z)

Examination Name	اسم الفحص
A	
Abdominal X-Ray	تصوير البطن بالأشعة السينية
Amniocentesis	بزل السلي / فحص ماء السلي / فحص السائل الأمينوزي
Alpha Fetoprotein Test (AFP)	فحص الزلال الجنيني
Allergy Skin Tests	اختبار حساسية الجلد
alanine transaminase	ناقلات الألانين
aldolase	إنزيم ألدولاز (aldolase)
Aldosterone test	تحليل الألدوستيرون
Audiometry	فحص السمع / قياس السمع
Auditory brainstem response (ABR)	فحص استجابة جذع المخ (ABR)
Alcohol level test	اختبار الكحول
Ambulatory E.C.G	تخطيط كهربيّة القلب السّامح بالتجوّل
Antibiotic susceptibility test	اختبار الاستعداد المناعي للمضادّات الحيويّة
Alkaline phosphatase	الفسفتاز القلوي
Amylase Test	تحليل الأميليز
Anti phospholipid antibody test	تحليل الأضداد المضادة للفوسفوليبيد
Antinuclear antibody	فحص الأجسام المضادة للنواة
Anti DNA antibody	أضداد ضد DNA
Anti smooth muscle antibody	الأجسام المضادة للعضلات الملساء
Anti glomerular basement membrane test	الأجسام المضادة لغشاء خلايا الكلى
Anti GAD ab test	تحليل أجسام مضادة موجهة ضد الإنزيم نازع كربوكسيل
Antithyroglobulin antibody	الأجسام المضادة للغدة الدرقية
Antithyroid microsomal antibody	الأجسام المضادة للجسيمات الصغيرة الدرقية
Anion gap	الفجوة الأنيونية ـ فجوة الصواعد
Arthroscopy	تنظير المفصل
Antidiuretic hormone test	الهرمون المضاد لإدرار البول
ACTH	الهرمون الموجه لقشر الكظر ACTH
Arterial blood gas	**غازات الدم الشرياني**
aspartate aminotransferase (GOT)	ناقلة أمين الأسبارتات (GOT)
Antistreptolysin O	**اختبار أضداد الحالة العقدية O**
Alpha -1 antitripsin test	فحص مضاد التربسين ألفا ـ 1
Angiotensin converting enzyme test	اختبار الإنزيم المحول للأنجيوتنسين
Amikacin level	أميكاسين
Aminophillin level	أمينوفيلين
B	
Blood Test	فحص الدم
Biopsy	الخزعة
Breast Biopsy	خزعة الثدي
Blood Pressure Check	قياس ضغط الدم
Bone Scan	تصوير العظام
Bone Mineral Density Test - DEXA	فحص هشاشة العظام DEXA
Blood chemistry	تحليل كيمياء الدم
Blood Calcium	الكالسيوم في الدم
Bone Marrow Biopsy	خزعة نخاع العظم
Blood Type Testing	فصيلة الدم

Blood culture	فحص زراعة الدم
Blood osmolality test	فحص الأسمولالية في الدم
Blood pH	درجة الحموضة
Bleeding time	زمن النزف
beta Human chorionic gonadotropin	موجهة الغدد التناسلية المشيمائية بيتا
bronchoscopy	تَنْظيرُ القَصَبات
Bender-Gestalt Test	اختبار بندر-جشطلت
Bilirubin test	تحليل البيليروبين
Biopsy of the vagina	خزعة المهبل
Breast ultrasound	تصوير الثدي بالموجات فوق الصوتية
Body fluid test	فحص سوائل الجسم

C

CMV Antibodies (Cytomegalovirus)	تحليل CMV الفيروس المُضَخِّم للخَلايا
CT - Computed Tomography	أشعة مقطعية ـ فحصCT
Chest X-Ray	تصوير الصدر
Complete Blood Count, CBC	فحص تعداد الدم CBC
Chorionic Villous Sampling, CVS	فحص الزغابات المشيمائية
Clotting Test	تجلط الدم
Colonoscopy, Sigmoidoscopy	تنظير القولون
Cardiac stress test	اختبار الجهد
Cholesterol and Triglycerides Test, Lipid Profile	اختبار الكوليسترول والدهون الثلاثية ، الدهون في الدم
CTG,CARDIO-TOCO-GRAPH,NST	مراقبة الجنين
Cystic Fibrosis Genetic Testing	فحص التليف الكيسي
Color vision test	اختبار عمى الألوان
chlamydia diagnostic tests	تحليل الكلاميديا
Cryoglobulin Blood Test	فحص الغلوبولينات البردية
Calcitonin test	فحص الكالسيتونين
Caloric stimulation	الاختبار الحَروري (لتحري وظيفة الدهليز بتقطير الماء الساخن في الصماخ الظاهر للأذن)
Cortisol test	فحص الكورتيزول
Coombs test	اختبار كومبس
Carboxyhemoglobin test	اختبار كربوكسي هيموغلوبين
Ceruloplasmin	فحص السيرولوبلازمين
Coronary catheterization	قسطرة القلب التشخيصية
Cystoscopy	تنظير المثانة
Cystometry	فحص قياس المثانة
CA - 125	فحص CA-125
Copper test	تحليل النحاس
Complement test	فحص المتممة
Corneal topography	تصوير القرنية
Chloride level test	نسبة الكلوريد في الدم
CRP test	اختبار البروتين المتفاعل C
Cold agglutinins blood test	فحص راصة دموية بردية
Cryptococcal antigen	مستضد المستخفيات
Carcinoembrionic antigen	المستضد السرطاني الجنيني
Creatinine blood test	فحص الكرياتينين
Creatine phosphokinase	فحص فسفوكيناز الكرياتين
Coagulation test	اختبارات التخثر
Colposcopy	تنظير المهبل

D	
D-xylose absorption test	اختبار امتصاص د-زايلوز
Diphenylhydantoin level	مستوى الهيدانتوين ثنائيُّ الفينيل
Dexamethasone supression test	اختبار كبت الديكساميثازون
Digoxin level	مستوى الديجوكسين
dehydroepiandrosterone sulfate	ديهيدرو إيبي أندروستيرون
Diagnosis of Angina Pectoris using Thallium Stress Test	تشخيص الذبحة الصدرية

E	
Echocardiogram	تخطيط صدى القلب
Erythrocyte Sedimentation Rate (ESR)	معدل ترسيب كريات الدم الحمراء
Esophago-gastro-duedenoscopy, Upper Endoscopy (EGD)	تنظير المعدة
Evoked potential test	اختبار الاستجابة المستثارة
Electronystagmography	تخطيط كهربية الرأراة
Electromyography – EMG	التخطيط الكهربائي للعضلات
Electroencephalography – EEG	التخطيط الكهربائي للدماغ - EEG
Electrocardiogram – ECG	تخطيط كهربية القلب
EKG	تخطيط كهربية القلب EKG
EBV antibodies test	تحليل أجسام مضادة لفيروس إبشتاين بار
Esophageal pH monitoring	مراقبة الحموضة في المريء
Estrogen Levels Test	تحليل هرمون الإستروجين
Endoscopic ultrasonography, Endoscopic ultrasound	تخطيط الصدى بالتنظير الداخلي
Electrophysiological testing of the conduction system	الاختبارات الفيزيولوجية الكهربائية للقلب
Electrocardiographic stress test	فحص تخطيط كهربيّة القلب خلال الجُهد

F	
Fetal Ultrasound	فحص أعضاء الجنين
Fragile X Testing	متلازمة كروموسوم x الهش
Fanconi's Anemia Testing	فقر الدم اللاتنسجي
Fetal Scalp pH Testing	فحص درجة حموضة فروة رأس الجنين
Familial dysautonomia	خلل الوظائف المستقلة العائلي
fibrinogen split products	نواتج انشطار الفيبرينوجين
Fundoscopy	تنظير قاع العين
Fluorescein angiography	تصوير قاع العين بعد حقن الفلوارسين Fluorescein
Fluorescein eye stain	صبغ العين بالفلورسين
Ferritin	فحص الفيرّيتين
Fibrinogen	تحليل الفيبرينوجين
Folic Acid	تحليل حمض الفوليك
follicle-stimulating hormone	هورمون منبه للجريب
Fetal blood test	فحص دم الجنين
Fetus sampling	الاعتيان الجنيني
Fetal position & Presentation	وضعية الجنين
Feces analysis	تحليل البراز
Fine Needle Localization (FNL)	تحديد موقع الورم بالإبرة الرفيعة

G

Glucose Test	فحص السكر
Gaucher's Disease Testing	فحص مرض غوشيه
Glucose tolerance test	اختبار تحمل الجلوكوز
Gallium scan	مسح الجاليوم
Growth Hormone Test	تحليل هرمون النمو
Gastrin hormone	هرمون الجاسترين
Gentamicin level	جنتاميسين
Glucose 6 phosphate dehydrogenase	إنزيم سداسي فوسفات الجلوكوز النازع للهيدروجين
Glucagon test	فحص الغلوكاغون
Globulin	الجلوبيولين
Gamma glutamyl transpeptidase test	فحص ناقلة الببتيد غاما غلوتاميل
Glucose Challenge Test	اختبار تحدي الجلوكوز
Genetic screening	تحليل الأمراض الوراثية
Gallium scan	تصوير الغاليوم
Gastric emptying scintigraphy	فحص تفريغ المعدة بواسطة التصوير الومضاني
Gastric bypass	المجازة المعدية

H

Hemoglobin Test	الهيموغلوبين
Heart Catheterization	قسطرة الشريان التاجي
Holter ECG	فحص هولتر – تخطيط كهربائية القلب المتنقل (لمراقبة نُظم القلب)
Hepatitis Test	تحليل التهاب الكبد
Herpes Virus Antibodies	تحليل الهربسpcr
Helicobacter pylori tests	الجرثومة الملوية البوابية
HIV test	تحليل الإيدز (نقص المناعة)
Hysterosalpingography	الأشعة الملونة للرحم
HIV resistance test	اختبار مقاومة فيروس نقص المناعة البشرية (HIV)
HIV viral load	حضانة فيروس نقص المناعة البشرية
Hepatitis A antibody test	تحليل التهاب الكبدA
Heterophil agglutination test	اختبار تراص غيروي
Hemoglobin A1C (Hb A1C)	السكر التراكمي / هيموغلوبين A1C
Homocysteine	تحليل الهوموسيستين
Haptoglobin	هابتوغلوبين
Head ultrasound in children	فحص رأس الأطفال بالأمواج فوق الصوتية
Hepatobiliary scan	المسح الكبدي الصفراوي
Histocompatibility Leucocyte Antigen	مستضد الكريات البيضاء البشرية

I

Iron Test	تحليل مخزون الحديد
Immunoelectrophoresis - IEP	فحص الرّحلان المناعي الكهربائي
Insulin resistance	تحليل مقاومة الإنسولين
Indocyanine green angiography (ICG)	تصوير قاع العين بعد حقنICG
IgM	أضداد من نوع IgM
IgG	أضداد من نوع IgG
IgE IE	أضداد من نوع IgE
IgA	أضداد من نوع IgA
Insulin antibody	مضاد الإنسولين

Intelligence quotient - IQ	اختبار الذكاء IQ
Intravenous urography	تصوير الحويضة الوريدية
Intravenous cholangiography	تصوير القنوات الصفراوية عن طريق الوريد
Imaging of the gastrointestinal tract	تصوير الجهاز الهضمي
Interventional radiology	التصوير الإشعاعي التدخّلي
Intestinal examination	فحص الأمعاء

K	اسم الفحص
Karyotype test	النمط النّووي
Kidney scan	تصوير الكلى
ketones urine test	تحليل الكيتونات في البول
Kidney Scan	تصوير الكلى بالنظائر المشعة
Kidney biopsy	خزعة الكلى

L	
LP - Lumbar Puncture	البَزْل القَطْنيّ
Liver Biopsy	خزعة الكبد
Liver Function Test	وظائف الكبد
Lymph Node Biopsy	خزعة العقد الليمفاوية
LE cell test	فحص الذئبة الحمامية
Lead test	فحص الرصاص
Lactose tolerance test	اختبار تحمل اللاكتوز
Liver and spleen scan	تصوير الكبد والطحال بالنظائر المشعة
Lithium	الليثيوم
lipase enzyme	أنزيم الليباز
Lactic dehydrogenase	نازع هيدروجين اللاكتات
Lactic acid	حمض اللاكتيك
luteinizing hormone	هرمون الملوتن
Lymphocytes (Lym)	اللمفاويات (Lym)
Lung function and challenge tests	اختبارات الأداء والتّحدّي التنفسي
Labeled WBC scintigraphy	التصوير الومضي لخلايا الدم البيضاء الموسومة
Lymphoscintigraphy	التصوير الومضاني الليمفاوي
Labeled red blood cells scintigraphy	التصوير الومضي بكريات الدم الحمراء الموسومة

M	
Mammography	التصوير الشعاعي للثدي
Magnetic Resonance Imaging - MRI	التصوير بالرنين المغناطيسي
Mean corpuscular volume, MCH, MCHC	حجم كريات الدم الحمراء
Mononucleosis Spot Test	اختبار كثرة الوحيدات العدوائية
Mantoux test	اختبار السل t
Manometry	قياس ضغط المريء
Magnesium	المغنيسيوم
Muscle Biops	خزعة العضل
Maternal blood screening in 1st and 2nd trimesters of pregnancy	تحرّي دم الأم في الثلث الأول والثاني من الحمل
MIBG scan	تصوير MIBG
Meckel's diverticulum scan	فحص تفريغ المعدة
Milk scan	فحص الحليب والأشعة

Manometry of the esoplagus and ano-rectum	قياس الضغط في المريء والشرج والمستقيم
Microscopic stool examination	فحص البراز المجهري

N	
Nuchal Translucency	الشفافية القفوية
Neutrophils, polymorphonuclears	العدلات (نوع من خلايا الدم البيض)
Natrium	صوديوم
Neutrophils (PMN)	العدلات
Nocturnal Penile Tumescence test	فحص الانتصاب الليلي
Nerve conduction study	اختبار توصيل العصب
Nuclear Cystography	تصوير المثانة بالنظائر المشعة

O	
O2 Saturation	درجة تشبع الأكسجين بالدم
Occult Blood Test	الدم الخفي في البراز
OGTT-Oral Glucose Challenge Test	تحمل الغلوكوز
otoacoustic emissions s	الانبعاث الصوتي من الأذن
Optical coherence tomography	التصوير المقطعي بالتماس البصري
Oxymetry	قياس مستوى تأكسج الدم
Octreotide scan	التصوير الومضاني لمستقبلات السوماتوستاتين
Open lung biopsy	الخزعة الرئوية المفتوحة

P	
Prostate specific antigen test	اختبار مستضد البروستاتا النوعي PSA
Pulmonary function tests	فحص وظائف الرئة
Pregnancy Test, Beta-hCG	اختبار الحمل Beta-hCG
Prostate Biopsy	فحص البروستاتا
Pap Smear, Papanicolaou Test	مسحة عنق الرحم
Polysomnogram	اختبار النوم
prolactin levels test	تحليل البرولاكتين
progesterone hormone test	تحليل هرمون البروجستيرون
phenylketonuria test	تحليل الفينيل كيتون يوريا
plasminogen	البلازمينوجين ـ مولد البلازمين
Porphyrins test	فحص البورفرينات
Paracetamol level	مستوى الباراسيتامول
positron emission tomography	التصوير المقطعي بالإصدار البوزيتروني
Plasma volume	فحص حجم البلازما
Phosphorus test	تحليل الفسفور
Partial thromboplastin time	اختبار زمن الترمبوبلاستين الجزئي
Prothrombin time	زمن البروثرومبين
Polymerase chain reaction	تفاعل سلسلة البوليميراز
Parathyroid Hormone Test	هرمون الغدة الجار درقية
Percutaneous cholangiography	تصوير القنوات الصفراوية عن طريق الجلد
Pulse	النبض
Prostate biopsy	خزعة البروستاتا
Potassium	البوتاسيوم
psychodiagnosis	الطب النفسي
Physical examination of the cardiovascular system	فحص القلب البدني
Psychogeriatric examination and evaluation	تقييم الحالة النفسية لكبار السن
Pelvic exam	الفحص الحوضي
PostCoital Test	فحص بعد الجماع
PET scan	التصوير المقطعي بالإصدار البوزيتروني

Q

Quick streptococcus A antigen test	فحص البكتيريا العقدية

R

Rubella Test	تحليل الحصبة الألمانية igG وigM
Reticulocytes	الخلايا الشبكية
Rorschach test	اختبار رورشاخ
Renin test	إنزيم الرنين
Radioactive iodine uptake test	فحص امتصاص اليود المشع
Radionuclide thyroid imaging	تصوير الغدة الدرقية بالنظائر المشعة
Rheumatoid factor	العامل الروماتويدي
Radionuclide scanning of the testis	تصوير الخصيتين بالأشعة
Rectal examination	فحص المستقيم

S

Semen Analysis	تحليل السائل المنوي
SPECT, PET , Heart Perfusion Scan, Cardiac blood pool scan ,MUGA Scan	فحص القلب بالنظائر المشعة
Screening Test	اختبار التقصي
Schilling Test	اختبار شيلينج
Serum cardiac biomarkers	علامات النوبة القلبية
Subjective Hearing Tests	اختبار السمع
Spinal Ultrasound	تصوير النخاع الشوكي بالموجات فوق الصوتية
Sinuses X-Ray	تصوير الوجه
Syphilis Antibodies	تحليل الزهري
Stool culture	زراعة البراز
Skin tests	اختبار الجلد
Schirmer's test	اختبار شيرمر
Sinus endoscopy	منظار الجيوب الانفية
Stress test	اختبار الإجهاد
Serotonin	السيروتونين
Sweat test	فحص التعرق
Short for endoscopic retrograde cholangiopancreatography	تصوير البنكرياس والقنوات الصفراوية بالتنظير الباطني بالطريق الراجع
Synovial biopsy	الخزعة الزليلية
SPECT scan	تصوير الدماغ الطبقي المحوسب بالانبعاث الأحادي الفوتون
Sigmoidoscopy	التنظير السيني

T

Throat Culture	مسحة الحلق
Tonometry (Intraocular Pressure Testing)	قياس ضغط العين
Testosterone Test	تحليل هرمون التستوستيرون
Toxoplasmosis Antibodies	فحص داء المقوسات
Test of Variables of Attention	اختبار تشتت الانتباه
TORCH screen test	فحصTORCH
Thyroxine - T4	فحص هرمون الغدة الدرقية
T helper	خلاياT
T supressor	الخلايا التائية
TIBC	القدرة على ربط الحديد بالترانسفيرين TIBC
Tissue typing	تنميط نسيجي
Thyroid Peroxidase Ab	أجسام مضادة للبيروكسيداز الدرقي
Transferrin	ترانسفيرين
Tryodothyronine	ثلاثي يود الثيرونين
Tensilon test	اختبار التنسيلون
Tympanometry	قياس الطبلة
Temperature test	قياس درجة الحرارة
Thyroid Stimulating Hormone (TSH)	فحص الهرمون المنبه للغدة الدرقية (TSH)
Tay-Sachs	تاي زاكس
Triglycerides (Trig)	فحص ثلاثي الغليسيريد
Transesophageal echocardiography	تخطيط صدى القلب عبر المريء
Tip toeing	استدقاق إصبع القدم
Tuberculin skin test	اختبار الجلد للكشف عن السل

Three-dimensional ultrasound in obstetrics and gynecology	الأشعة فوق الصوتية ثلاثي الأبعاد/ طب النّساء
Thyroid gland imaging	تصوير الغدة الدرقية
Testis US	فحص الخصية بالأمواج فوق الصوتية

U	
Urine test	فحص البول
Urine culture	مزرعة البول
Ultrasound	الموجات فوق الصوتية
Urobilinogen	يوروبيلينوجين
Urinanalysis	تحليل البول
Urine toxicology screen	تحليل المخدرات في البول
Urea	فحص اليوريا Urea
Ultrasound in pregnancy	التصوير بالأشعة فوق الصوتيّة عند الحمل
Ultrasound, Fetal biometry	التصوير فوق الصوتي لقياس عمر الجنين
Ultrasound of the urinary tract in children	فحص المسالك البولية لدى الأطفال بالأمواج فوق الصوتية
Ultrasound of abdomen and pelvis	فحص البطن والحوض بواسطة الأمواج فوق الصوتية
US - Doppler of carotid arteries	تصوير الأوردة بالأمواج فوق الصوتية للشرايين السباتية
Ultrasound - doppler of veins	فحص دوبلر (الأمواج فوق الصوتية)
Urodynamic evaluation	فحص ديناميكا البول
Urodynamics study	فحص ديناميكا البول

V	
Virtual Colonoscopy	التنظير القولوني الافتراضي
Video Capsule Endocopy, VCE	تنظير الجهاز الهضمي
Ventilation-Perfusion Scan	تصوير الرئتين بالنظائر المشعة
Visual Field Test - Perimetry Test	فحص مجال الرؤية
Vitamin B12 Testing	تحليل فيتامين ب12
Venography	تصوير الأوردة
Very low density lipoproteins test	فحص البروتينات الدهنية منخفض الكثافة جدّا
Visual acuity test	اختبار النظر

W	
WBC	كريات الدم البيضاء
West - Nile Virus Test	فحص حمى النيل الغربي

X	
X-Ray	التصوير بالأشعة السينية
Xylose tolerance test	اختبار تحمل الزايلوز

Z	
Zinc level	فحص الزنك

- **Vitamin and Minerals**

Vitamin and Minerals	اسم الفيتامين أو المعدن
Folic acid	حمض الفوليك (فيتامين ب9)
Vitamin B6	فيتامين ب6
Vitamin A	فيتامين أ (الرتينول)
Vitamin B5	فيتامين ب 5
vitamin B1	فيتامين ب1 (الثيامين)
Vitamin B12	فيتامين ب12 (الكوبالامين)
vitamin B2	فيتامين ب2 (الريبوفلافين)
Vitamin B3	فيتامين ب3 (النياسين)
Vitamin H	فيتامين ب7
Vitamin C	فيتامين ج (حمض الأسكوربيك)
Vitamin D	فيتامين د
Vitamin K	فيتامين ك
Vitamin E	فيتامين هـ
Potassium	معدن البوتاسيوم
Ferrus	معدن الحديد
Zinc	معدن الزنك
Selenium	معدن السيلينيوم
Sodium	معدن الصوديوم
Fluoride	معدن الفلورايد
Calcium	معدن الكالسيوم
Chromium	معدن الكروم
Magnesium	معدن المغنيسيوم (المغنيزيوم)
Copper	معدن النحاس
Iodine	معدن اليود

Section 3

REALISTIC SCENARIOS AT HOSPITALS

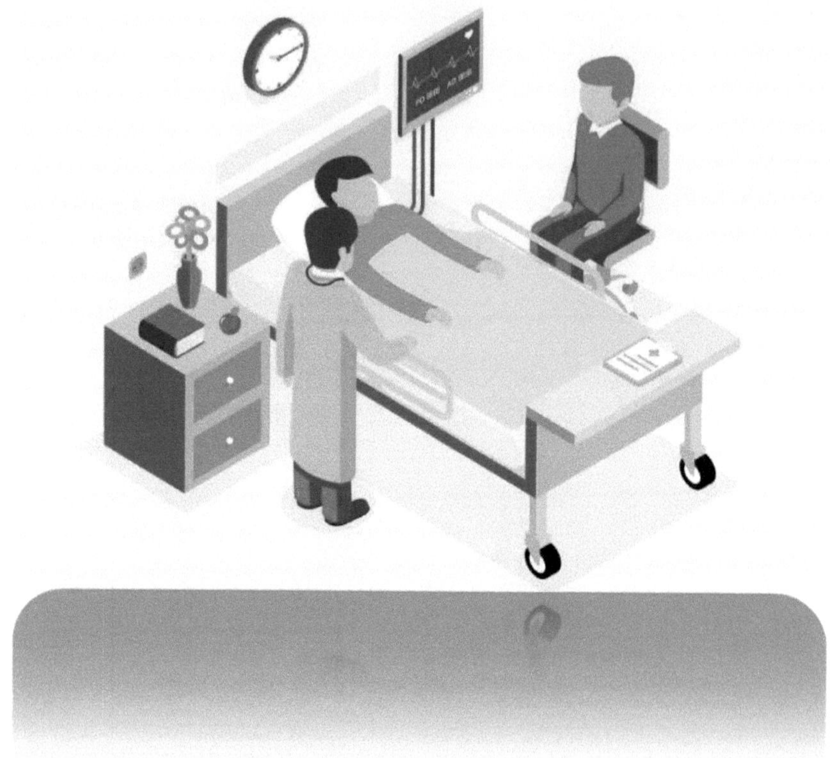

تعبّر السيناريوهات التالية عن محاكاة للواقع من المستشفيات في أي مكان في العالم.

وجميع الشخصيات والأحداث من وحي خيال المؤلف ، وأي تشابه مع الأشخاص

أو الأحداث الحقيقية هو من قبيل الصدفة البحتة.

These are simulated scenarios from hospitals anywhere in the world.

All the characters and events are fictitious, and any similarity to actual people

or events is purely coincidental.

Script 1	Post-endoscopy
Physician	If you would let her know the first thing we're going to do, to do some questions and brief medical assessment to get her ready for her procedure
Interpreter	
LEP	نعم
Interpreter	
Physician	This is Dr James and here is the Arabic interpreter, How do you feel now?
Interpreter	
LEP	الحمد لله , زين الحين بس في عوار في البطن شويه
Physician	This is usual thing happen after the procedure. I'm here to tell you that you prep. Very well, before the procedure.
Interpreter	
Physician	The procedure has been achieved very well, I did find 3 polyps
LEP	تمام
Interpreter	
Physician	I have removed them, they were 2 mm in diameter, I am not worried about
Interpreter	
Physician	We have sent the specimen to laboratory, and once we get results, I'll let you know
Interpreter	
Physician	It's benign polyps, that no worries.
Interpreter	
LEP	تمام
Interpreter	
Physician	You need to repeat the procedure within 1 year
Interpreter	

Script 2	General Surgery Clinic – Postop Colonoscopy follow-up
Physician	Today, your 1 week follow-up post colonoscopy
Interpreter	
LEP	نعم, صحيح
Interpreter	
Physician	As I told you earlier that we found 2 polyps in the colon and that has been removed and sent to pathology, and good news that they were benign.
Interpreter	
LEP	طيب الحمد لله
Physician	You need to repeat the procedure within 1 year, as your Prep. Was insufficient.
Interpreter	
LEP	يعني متى يا دكتور, الأولاد في مدارس واحنا من مكان بعيد, هل ممكن نسويه في شهر 10
Interpreter	
Physician	Within year, means next week or any day before one year, so October will b this time ok
LEP	تمام يا دكتور كويس اسويه في اكتوبر قبل بداية امتحانات المدارس
Interpreter	
Physician	You need to have good prep. This time.
Interpreter	
LEP	والله المره اللي طافت ما أكلت لمدة يومين, وشربت ماي كتير, مع الشراب اللي اعطيهوني, بس الشراب كان متعب ويسبب لوعة, كل 10 دقايق, أوقف واشرب ثاني
Physician	This time you need to drink enough water, and I will double the dose of laxative drink
Interpreter	
LEP	يا دكتور ده بيسبب لوعة, الشراب هذا
Interpreter	
Physician	This nausea is something normal after taking the syrup
Interpreter	
LEP	هل ممكن تبدل الشراب بشيء ثاني أقوى
Physician	I will add some tablets with the syrup, that will help
Interpreter	
LEP	مشكور يا دكتور, ممكن تشرح لي ثاني هو ايه كان النتوء ده , يعني مش سرطان
Interpreter	
Physician	Benign polyps are the opposite of cancer ones.
Interpreter	
LEP	أصل أنا كان عندي نتوء قبل كده في الرحم, المبيض, وجزء من الأمعاء, والطبيب خبرني وقتها انه سرطان وتم استئصاله
Physician	I was not aware of that last visit, are you sure the polyps on the ovaries were cancer
Interpreter	
LEP	نعم كان النتوء أو الورم هذا في المبايض وكان سرطاني وتم استئصال المبيض الأيسر وترك الأيمن
Physician	If it was cancerous one, he should have removed the two ovaries.
Interpreter	
LEP	خبرني الطبيب انه المبيض الأيمن فيه جزء صغير وأفضل نشيل الايسر فقط, عشان ازالة المبيضين يسبب اضطراب في الهرمونات وترهلات في الجسم
Interpreter	

Physician	Ok, I understand, but I think it was not cancerous, let me ask did the surgeon have removed the left ovary and uterus in one session, and let's schedule you for the procedure in October
Interpreter	
LEP	ايوه يا دكتور في نفس العملية شال الرحم والمبيض الأيسر, هل في أدوية الحين لازم أخدها
Interpreter	
Physician	No need for medication now, just collect the syrup from pharmacy and follow instruction slip that nurse will give, to start good prep. Before the procedure next time.
Interpreter	
LEP	مشكورة يا دكتور, ما قصرت
Interpreter	

Script 3	Pulmonary Clinic –Initial Consultation – Apnea
Physician	What are your suffering from today
LEP	أحيانا وأنا نايم باحسن ان نفسي بينقطع, وحرقان في الرئة لازم أصحى اشرب ماي عشان وجع الصدر يروح, ولو ما شربت الوجع يزيد
Interpreter	
Physician	Does your sneezing disturb your sleeping?
LEP	على طول بينشيني من النوم
Interpreter	
Physician	Are you kicking while sleeping?
LEP	لا
Interpreter	
Physician	Are you speaking while sleeping?
LEP	لا الحمد لله طبيعي
Physician	Are you walking while sleeping?
LEP	لا الحمد لله ما وصلنا للمرحلة دي
Physician	Are you allergic to any medications? And have you undergone any surgeries in the past?
Interpreter	
LEP	لا ما في حساسية, بس سويت عملية قص معدة
Interpreter	
Physician	Are you thinking of another gastric surgery?
Interpreter	
LEP	نعم, عندي موعد اليوم مع جراح السمنة عشان اسوي تغيير مسار, وميعاد مع أخصائية التغذية
Interpreter	
Physician	When was your previous gastric sleeve surgery?
Interpreter	
LEP	من اربع سنوات
Interpreter	
Physician	Now we are going to do breathing test and to schedule for sleep study
Interpreter	
LEP	يعني اسوي الفحص الحين, طيب وايش يعني دراسة النوم هذه, يعني هاتنوم بالمستشفى
Physician	Yes, sleep study, you will come one day in the evening sleep in the hospital, next day morning you will be discharged,
Interpreter	
Physician	Then once we receive results, I'll explain plan of treatment.
Interpreter	
LEP	مشكور يا دكتور

Script 4	Rheumatology Clinic –follow-up
Physician	Today is your due date for osteoporosis injection, and I'll refill the supplements
Interpreter	
LEP	تمام يا دكتور, يعني فيتامين د, والحديد والدم زين
Interpreter	
Physician	Your vitamin D is good, but you need to maintain taking the vitamin D tablet, once a week, and inflammatory factor is getting lower., that something is good.
Interpreter	
LEP	طيب انت خبرتني قبل كده ان فيتامين د, أخده مره واحدة كل شهر, وهل الروماتيزم تبعي على المدى البعيد ممكن يخرب حاجات تانية في الجسم
Interpreter	
Physician	This dose that once monthly was 50,000 mmg, now the dose of vitamin D is 10,000mg once a week is more than enough, and regarding your rheumatoid as long as we repeat blood test every month, no further damage could be caused by rheumatoid to the body. So today we'll repeat blood test
Interpreter	
LEP	مشكور يا دكتور طمنتني
Physician	Now your son need to collect the medication from the pharmacy for the injection, I placed the order on the system, then you will receive the injection
LEP	الله يحفظك يا دكتور
Interpreter	

Physician	What are you complaining and symptoms?
Interpreter	
LEP	عندي ضيق في التنفس, بعد ما أصبت بكورونا, وعاوزه أطمن على الرئة عشان اشوف اخذ التطعيم بتاع الكورونا ولا لا
Interpreter	
Physician	When have you exposed to covid?
Interpreter	
LEP	من شهر تقريبا, وتم حجري بالفندق وبعد ما طلعت راجعت الدكتور وخبرني اني لازم اخد اكسجين عشان ذار عندي التصاق في الشعب الهوائية
Interpreter	
Physician	Did you take oxygen in the hotel, and for how long are you taking the oxygen
Interpreter	
LEP	في الفندق ما اخذت اكسجين بس خدته لما طلعت ولمدة اسبوع واحد ووقفته
Interpreter	
Physician	Why did you stop oxygen?
Interpreter	
LEP	سوى لي ضيق في النفس ووجع على الصدر
Physician	Are you allegoric to any food, medication
Interpreter	
LEP	عندي حساية من الغبرة, العطور, ومن جميع المضادات الحيوية والانسولين, احنا عندنا بالعيلة سكري من الدرجة الأولى مع أي انسولين بيحصل حساسية
Interpreter	
Physician	Now we will send you to do chest xray and breathing test, the I'll see you again to discuss the findings and plan of treatment
Interpreter	
LEP	مشكور
Interpreter	

Script 6	Spine Clinic – follow-up
Physician	How are you today? And how is your pain level compared to last visit
Interpreter	
LEP	نشكر الله على كل حال, بس الوجع بقى بينزل من أسفل الظهر على الرجل, وما باقدر انام بالليل بسبة الوجع
Interpreter	
Physician	Is you lower back pain radiating to right or left legs, and where posterior, lateral, medial And till where the pain radiate till ankle, knee or foot
Interpreter	
LEP	العوار بينزل على الرجل اليسار اكثر وبعض الاحيان اليمين, وبيكون على اليسار من ورا الفخذ وينزل لي التبانة من ورا لحد الكاحل, وساعات بيكون فيه تنميل وعنان ووخز
Interpreter	
Physician	Is the numbness constant or in and off, and for how long did start?
LEP	التنميل مستمر وبيزيد بالليل وقت الرقاد, وبقاله شهر تقريبا
Interpreter	
Physician	Today I will review the MRI that you have underwent 10 days ago, it shows that you have herniated disc between L4 - L5 THAT compressing the nerve on the left side that is moderate. And as well protrusion between L1, L2, L3 but just mild one
Interpreter	
LEP	يعني انفتاق الديسك هذا هو اللي مسبب لي العوار والتنميل اللي بين الرابعة والخامسة
Interpreter	
Physician	Yes L4-L5 causing the symptoms you have on legs We need to start with physiotherapy for one month and if no improvement you will need a surgery called OLM (Open Lumbar Microdiscectomy)
Interpreter	
LEP	مشكور يا دكتور
Physician	Can I do now physical assessment , during the assessment if you start to have any pain or symptom, please do let me know on spot
Interpreter	
LEP	حاضر يا دكتور أنام على ضهري الحين
Interpreter	
Physician	yes, raise your right ankle up, more and more, I want to see your power, is there any pain
Interpreter	
LEP	في عوار بسيط في أسفل الظهر قبل العصعص على الطرف اليسار
Interpreter	
Physician	Where I touch here is there any pain
Interpreter	
Physician	Now can you start to walk on your tip toes, and take off your slippers
Interpreter	
LEP	لا، زين يا دكتور, بس اخاف اطيح
Interpreter	
Physician	Don't worry, I will help you
LEP	تمام

Interpreter	
Physician	Now you need to go to reception to schedule your physio and follow-up after one month
LEP	كم مرة العلاج الطبيعي بالاسبوع
Interpreter	
Physician	Twice a week plus let them teach you some home exercises to do at home
LEP	دكتور ممكن اروح الجيم, والعب كرة قدم ولا ده ممنوع الحين
Interpreter	
Physician	Just fast walking is op, please refrain from lifting any heavyweight above your shoulder, that will make more compression on the disc
Interpreter	
LEP	مشكور
Interpreter	

Physician	I just want to verify that your appointment for today is for physical
Interpreter	
LEP	نعم
Interpreter	
Physician	Any allergies to any food, or medicines that you know of
Interpreter	
LEP	لا
Physician	Have you traveled out the country within the last 30 days
Interpreter	في شهر مارس العام الماضي
Physician	Have you been recently in the emergency room or hospitalized?
LEP	في بداية السنة
Interpreter	
Physician	How are you preventing pregnancy, do you use male condom, or not sexually active, or you do rely on your partner?
Interpreter	
Physician	Do you currently smoke or did you previously tobacco
Interpreter	
Physician	Do you drink any alcohol,
Interpreter	
LEP	
Interpreter	
Physician	Just to confirm your primary care doctor is dr. Michael
Interpreter	Pharmacy is WS in the main street
LEP	I am gonna take your vital s really quick and take blood pressure
Interpreter	
Physician	Can you let me know, it's possible that the doctor checks your feet today?
Interpreter	
	You are due soon for a colon cancer screening, isnot it?
	If we give you a stool kit to have
	Have you received the flu shot for this year for the month of August

Physician	The baby is for Tylenol 1.4 ml., and I'll send that over to pharmacy and he can have the next dose after 06.20 tonight if he needs it.
Interpreter	
LEP	
Interpreter	
Physician	I have already gone over all instructions for the Vaseline and every diaper change. And everything I have is checkup and postop his procedure on Monday 11 November at 9 o'clock in the morning.
LEP	
Physician	Let me check his diaper really quick, everything looks good. It's going to be red and swollen but everything looks how it's supposed to be right now.
Interpreter	
Physician	Do you have any questions about anything?
LEP	
Interpreter	
Physician	Okay, is that from mom's feeding him
Interpreter	
Physician	We know that happens sometimes from mom feeding
Interpreter	
Physician	You don't have to check out or anything when youre ready you are good to go
Interpreter	

Physician	They did upper stretch of his esophagus and they also stretched part of his stomach
Interpreter	
LEP	
Interpreter	
Physician	They stretched with the balloon, that's how we spread.
Interpreter	
LEP	
Physician	They stretch it with the balloon and then they inflate the balloon and take the balloon out but it looks like it was stretched out good
Interpreter	
Physician	They stretched out the throat as well and they did a camera down the throat so everything looked okay from that side, there is no cancer or tumors or anything.
LEP	
Interpreter	
Physician	So sometimes it can come back, but we will see how he feels with the stretched that they did today and they keep in close contact with you guys to see how he is feeling and everything after this procedure today
Interpreter	
Physician	There was a tube that was brought down, but it was the camera brought down and they did a stretch with a different kind of cylinder that helps stretch out upper throat and everything.
Interpreter	
Physician	Any further questions
Interpreter	
LEP	

Physician	You had car accident, and got some fractures and bruises on your body
Interpreter	
LEP	مش متذكر, اخر شيئ اتذكره كنت راكب السيارة مع زوجتي وبعد كده, أتذكر ان في 4 افراجد كسروا باب السيارة واخدومي بالاسعاف
Interpreter	
Physician	You have been taken to The city hospital, because you have fractures on rib no 3 thru 7, and pubic area fractures, bruises around right kidney, and lungs as well
Interpreter	
LEP	هل وضعي الصحي خطير, كمني يا دكتور
Physician	To be honest, you have been shifted from the other hospital to this hospital for hospitalization and observation, we need to make sure that the bruises are not getting bigger in size, and healing well.
Interpreter	
LEP	يعني هاعمل اشعة ولا اية بالظبط,
Interpreter	
Physician	You had done x-rays, and now we will do CT to check if there is any damage around heart and its function
LEP	احب اعرفك يا دكتور ان نسيت اخد برشام الضغط الصبح, وحاولت اجرب ادخل الحمام ما عرفت اتبول كتير, لان الحبة كانت بتساعد على ادرار البول
Interpreter	
Physician	Do you have any urine incontinence or any other symptoms
Interpreter	
LEP	ساعة الحادث كان في ألم كثير تحت لمؤاخذ في منطقة الخصية, بس دلوقتي احسن, بس في ألم مطان عملية فتاق البطن, خايف ليكون فتح تاني
Physician	We will do some scanning and to rest assured everything is ok
Interpreter	
LEP	بس محتاج اعمل حمام ومش عارف
Interpreter	
Physician	We will give some diuretic to help with, but be careful because you have some injury on left leg, you need assistance from nurse to help when you want to urinate
Interpreter	
LEP	احب اعمل الحمام وانا واقف ده هيساعد البول يخرج, بس الموضوع محرج ان ممرضة تكون معايا, هاخلي ابني يساعدني وانا واقف
Physician	It's ok as long as someone assist you
Interpreter	
LEP	مشكور يا دكتور, ممكن تشرح لي تاني هو ممكن اخرج امتى من المستشفى
Interpreter	
Physician	After observation and to ensure that your vitals and injuries are getting better you can can get discharged, but you have some serious injuries bruises and fractures that need to be to looked after medically, before going home
Interpreter	
LEP	ربنا يحفظك ويخليك يا اكتور على المساعدة والاهتمام
Physician	We are here to help you and take care of you, by the way your wife got injuried as well but her condition is stable
Interpreter	
LEP	شكرا يا دكتور

Physician	I'd like to tell you that my name is Dr Sally, one of the doctors from the medical team, taking care of Mr. Ahmed
Interpreter	
LEP	مرحبا، أهلا وسهلا
Interpreter	
Physician	So we admit Mr. Ahmed because he has cellulites of his right butt. Cellulites basically means that he has an infection of his skin, that's why we admitted him, so in cellulites we have to give IV antibiotics right now
Interpreter	
LEP	يعني محتاج ابقى هنا بالمشفى ولمدة كم يوم؟
Physician	So right now, we think he should need antibiotic at least for five to seven days, but we have infectious disease specialists who are also seeing him. They saw him this morning so we will talk to them and to find out how many days they want the antibiotic to be running. But you know, most likely five to seven days but he doesn't need to stay in the hospital that long, you know we can once he starts getting better to transfer the IV antibiotic to oral by mouth, but because he sis still sick we will keep him at least for today and see him tomorrow to see how he feels
Interpreter	
LEP	ممكن أفهم ايه التشخيص بالظبط لأني ما فهمت شي من الحكي
Interpreter	
Physician	It's called cellulites, it is usually infection of your skin and the tissue that is underneath the skin, so the skin or the soft tissue that is beneath the skin has infection. Different things that can cause it most, you know, most commonly if you hit yourself or there's an injury or trauma in anywhere, then that can cause cellulites and some people if they take injection that can cause cellulites as well. So right now we don't know the cause
LEP	ممكن اخرج اليوم على البيت، محتاج اروح, حاسس اني كويس الحين, ممكن؟
Interpreter	
Physician	For at least for now, for today, we'll keep him in the hospital, you know, because he still has some pain and we are giving him IV antibiotiic. So today we cannot send him home. He has to stay tomorrow, we will see him again and how he is doing, if he looks okay, we will examine his butt to ensure no abcess or redness, swelling that we will think about discharging him.
Interpreter	
LEP	مشكور يا دكتورة، أمرنا لله

Script 12	GI Clinic
Physician	Your vital sign looks great, blood pressure 102/70 is normal
Interpreter	
LEP	الحمد لله, ربنا يطمنك
Interpreter	
Physician	Have you done any surgeries in the past, and are you taking any medicine right now
Interpreter	
LEP	سويت عملية اللوز في بلدي, وباخد دوا السكر والضغط وأدوية تانية مش فاكراها
Physician	So only tonsillectomy nothing else, ok, you can give me your pharmacy number to call to get list of medicine
Interpreter	
LEP	متى هاشوف الدكتور
Interpreter	
Physician	The doctor is going to see you shortly, just wait in here
LEP	مشكورة يا حبيبتي
Interpreter	
Physician	Hello, how are you?, my name is dr. Donald, your GI doctor, Your doctor has sent over some paperwork that I read through. But I'd like to hear from you first what is going on?
Interpreter	
LEP	بص بقى يا دكتور, أنا باعاني من جرثومة المعدة من 4 أو 5 شهور ودكتوري السابق عمل كذا منظار, وكل مرة يقول عندي جرثومة, ويعطيني كورس علاج, امشي عليه والجرثومة ما بتروح, تعبت من الموضوع واللي خلاني أخاف اكثر ان الدكتور كان بيقول الجرثومة من غير علاج ممكن تسبب سرطان, عشان كده حببت اغير الدكتور
Physician	I see, when is your last endoscopy, and last time you were positive for H-pylori
Interpreter	
LEP	شهر 3 على ما افتكر وساعتها كان عندي جرثومة, عشان عاوزة ابدأ على بياض معاك ونعرف ايه المشكلة وليه العلاج ما بيشتغل ويخلصني من الجرثومة, انا تعبت كتير والله, وباذن الله الشفا على ايدك
Interpreter	
Physician	So what we can do now is to start with repeating EGD, that's for reasons, first of all to confirm if that was the right diagnosis, second, if H-pylori still there or not, third if there is anything else causing trouble
Interpreter	
LEP	يعني ما ينفعش نبدأ بالتصوير والأشعة قبل المنظار لانه متعب
Physician	I prefer to start with EGD other than scanning, as it's much quicker, to give us an idea of what is going on, then everything is ok with endoscopy, we will move forward with some scanning, then give the right medicine, but if it's positive, we would give stronger medicine that I believe you did not try before
Interpreter	
LEP	حاضر يا دكتور يا عسل أنت, والله ارتاحت لك, ربنا يبارك فيك, امتى هاعمل المنظار, ياريت بسرعة بس مش يوم الأحد عشان باروح الكنيسة, ومش بدري أوي عشان باوصل الأولاد على المدارس
Interpreter	
Physician	I'll let the scheduler come and schedule your EGD and I said no prep needed for this procedure, just no food or during from mid night as I mentioned, and we'll request authorization from insurance before proceeding, then will let you know if there is any rejection from insurance
Interpreter	

LEP	شكرا, ربنا يخليك, ويجعل على ايدك الشفا، معلش كنت عماله أتكلم كتير
Physician	No worries
Interpreter	

Script 13	GI Clinic
Physician	Hey, based on ultrasound, your kidney, liver are okay, except gallbladder, you do have stones
Interpreter	
LEP	يعني هل الحالة خطيرة يا دكتور
Interpreter	
Physician	Some people live with gallbladder without any symptoms or need of surgery, in your case I'll refer you to surgeon to discuss further
Interpreter	
LEP	الطبيب السابق كان قال شيئ على المبيض بس مش فاكرة ايه كانت المشكلة
Physician	No ovarian cyst, but you have little infection in urine that need antibiotic treatment
Interpreter	
LEP	يعني محتاجة عملية
Interpreter	
Physician	You don't need surgery, but if symptoms getting worse or having fever you need to come back here

Physician	My name is Dr. Peter, this is Dr. Johnson and we're a couple of the supervising doctor, let us know what's been going on with your daughter?
Interpreter	
LEP	تقريبا من سنتين، ترجع، تطرش، تدوخ، وبطنها توجعها، والتهاب في البول
Interpreter	
Physician	This has been going on for two years
Interpreter	
LEP	تيجي وتروح, نسعفها في الطواريء؛ بطنها توجعها، دوخة, صداع، وتاخد اجازات من المدرسة كل أسبوعين، وتشخيصهم الدائم: التهاب في المثانة والزائدة الدودية
Physician	Tell us about the vomiting like how often is she throwing up? What is she throwing up?
Interpreter	
LEP	أيام أيام، المدرسة تتصل بنتكم تقول بتتقيؤ، وعاوزة ترجع البيت، يعني في الصباح تكون كويسة في المدرسة تتقيؤ 3-4 مرات, وتغيب عن المدرسة
Interpreter	
Physician	All right, why did you bring her in today? Like if this has been going on for two years now, what's changed? I guess in the last day or so that said you bring her into the ER.
LEP	عشان نسعفها للطواريء الأقرب للبيت، لأن اليوم في صداع عاوزين نطمن على دماغها، وزمان كان عندها دم بالبول
Interpreter	
Physician	Did you guys try anything at home? Did you guys give her any medications at home
Interpreter	
LEP	استخدمت مضاد حيوي من 3 أيام خلصته, وده كان موصوف من أسبوعين
Physician	That what was that for?
Interpreter	
LEP	قالوا انها عندها التهابات في الزائدة
Interpreter	
Physician	All right and then tell me about like so obviously she is vomiting now, is she having any diarrhea? Any fevers that she's had at home, like anything that you guys have measured at home
Interpreter	
LEP	مفيش اسهال، ولا كانت بتحمى في البيت
Physician	How is she eating and drinking?
Interpreter	
LEP	ضعيف الشهية
Interpreter	
Physician	So we are going to take a quick feel at her belly here and then we can kind of come up with a plan
Interpreter	
LEP	حاضر
Physician	So dad and mom, we are gong to have to do a pretty workout, okay? So I'm gonna swab her throat to check for strep because strep throat can cause these symptoms of a headache, the belly pain, throwing off, can cause all these things, so that is the first thing, and then when she has to go pee, we would like her to pee into the cup to check if she has urinary tract infection

Interpreter	
Physician	Then in addition to the urine and the swab, we're also going to get some blood work and then a picture of her belly.
LEP	
Physician	If there is no any questions or concerns right now? I think we are all set.

<table>
<tr><td colspan="2">Script 15</td></tr>
<tr><td>Physician</td><td>I am returning your call, how may I help you?</td></tr>
<tr><td>Interpreter</td><td></td></tr>
<tr><td>LEP</td><td dir="rtl">أنا قررت خلاص اني اولد طبيعي</td></tr>
<tr><td>Interpreter</td><td></td></tr>
<tr><td>Physician</td><td>If this is your decision we can schedule you for the pre-op on Monday 6 Feb, at the burger building, to do blood work, and the very next day the induction of labor</td></tr>
<tr><td>Interpreter</td><td></td></tr>
<tr><td>LEP</td><td dir="rtl">يعني هاولد يوم الأثنين</td></tr>
<tr><td>Physician</td><td>No, it's just preparation and directions of the labor, the induction will take place the next day either am or am at your convenient</td></tr>
<tr><td>Interpreter</td><td></td></tr>
<tr><td>LEP</td><td dir="rtl">خليها الصبح الساعة 10 ، ممكن اعرف هتاخد اد ايه الولادة, وهل هتعطوني بقايا المولود</td></tr>
<tr><td>Interpreter</td><td></td></tr>
<tr><td>Physician</td><td>We will start the labor induction on Tuesday 10am, and we will not hurry the process, so we don't know how long is going to take, it depends, and in regards the remains, we will give it funeral house not you.</td></tr>
<tr><td>LEP</td><td dir="rtl">يعني مش هاخد بقايا المولود</td></tr>
<tr><td>Interpreter</td><td></td></tr>
<tr><td>Physician</td><td>You will take it from funeral home, as there is process to follow, issue death certificate, give remains, signing in some paperwork,…</td></tr>
<tr><td>Interpreter</td><td></td></tr>
<tr><td>LEP</td><td dir="rtl">يعني مينفعش ناخد البيبي علطول بدل ال funeral ده</td></tr>
<tr><td>Physician</td><td>Unfortunately , no we must follow the process</td></tr>
<tr><td>Interpreter</td><td></td></tr>
<tr><td>LEP</td><td dir="rtl">طيب هياخد وقت عشان يعطونا البيبي, عشان ندفنه بسرعة في مدافن المسلمين</td></tr>
<tr><td>Interpreter</td><td></td></tr>
<tr><td>Physician</td><td>I'll provide the all information at that time to check with them how long is going to take</td></tr>
<tr><td>Interpreter</td><td></td></tr>
<tr><td>LEP</td><td dir="rtl">هل بيبقى في صعوبات مع ولادة طفل ميت</td></tr>
<tr><td>Physician</td><td>It depends and it's same complication like any other delivery, we will monitor everything while you are in labor induction, don't worry too much.</td></tr>
<tr><td>Interpreter</td><td></td></tr>
<tr><td>LEP</td><td dir="rtl">هل الولادة هتكون في بناية burger ولا فين</td></tr>
<tr><td>Interpreter</td><td></td></tr>
<tr><td>Physician</td><td>No, the main hospital 3rd floor</td></tr>
<tr><td>Interpreter</td><td></td></tr>
</table>

INTERACTIVE GAMES AND CROSSWORD

Medical Terminology Quiz

Your medical interpretation career will flourish if you master it.

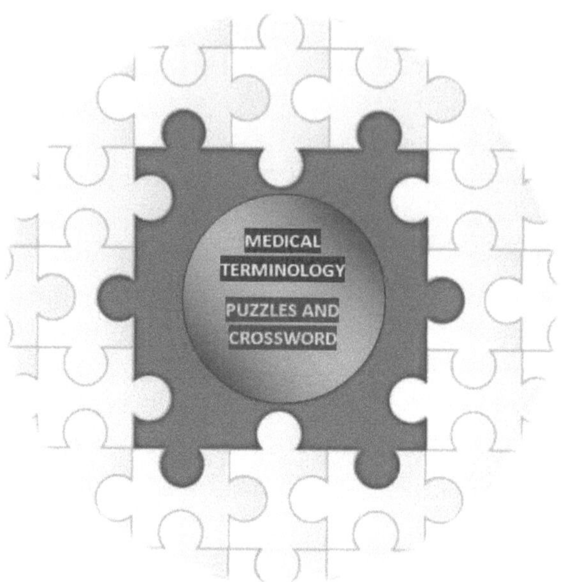

Overview

The purpose of this part of the book is to help you, practice what you learned in medical terminology, making it more enjoyable for you and more focused on the subject.

Our quizzes are designed to help you learn the language of medicine as frequently as you need to.

- Crosswords
- Fill in blanks
- Multiple choice questions
- Who am I?
- Answer key

We hope you enjoy answering quizzes and puzzles

During the learning process, repetition is a vital component.

*The Answer Keys Are Available At The End Of The Quiz.

Crossword

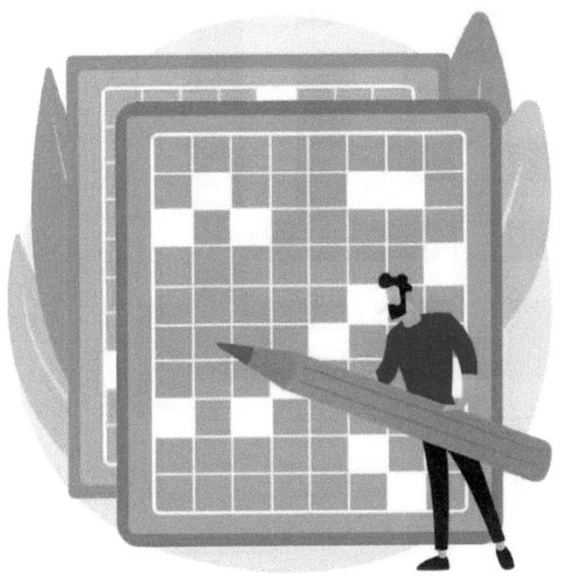

- **Crossword puzzle no. 1**

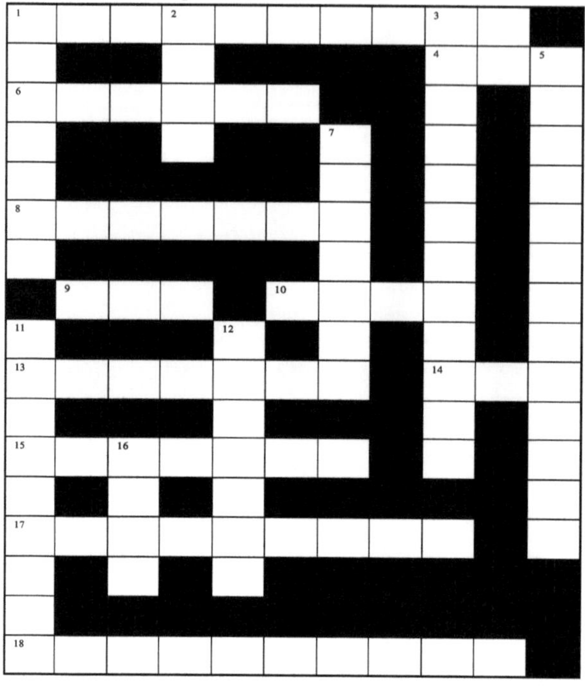

<u>Clues</u>

Across

1. A disease or abnormality present from birth (10 letters)

4. (Acronym) Symptoms women can get before their period (3 letters)

6. A suffix meaning suture or surgical repair (6 letters)

8. A type of seizure that causes you to blank out for a few seconds (7 letters)

9. Common word for feeling sick or unwell (3 letters)

10. An essential trace mineral needed for growth, DNA synthesis, immune function, etc. (4 letters)

13. The wasting away of body tissue or an organ (7 letters)

14. Coconut, Olive, canola and fish are all healthy examples of this (3 letters)

15. To insert or fix an artificial object in a person's body, especially by surgery (7 letters)

17. Inflammation of the tonsils that causes sore throat and pain when swallowing (11 letters)

18. Nerve damage that causes pain, weakness, numbness and/or tingling (10 letters)

Down

1. Relating to the heart (7 letters)
2. Acronym for a genetic disorder that causes red blood cells to break down when exposed to certain triggers
3. Surgical removal of the appendix (12 letters)
5 . A small fracture between two vertebrae, also called pars defect (13 letters)
7. A condition involving having too much body fat (7 letters)
11. Waves of energy that can penetrate tissue and can be used to diagnose or treat diseases (9 letters)
12. Failure of an organ or tissue to develop or to function normally (7 letters)
16. The part of your brainstem that handles unconscious processes like sleep-wake cycle and breathing (4 letters)

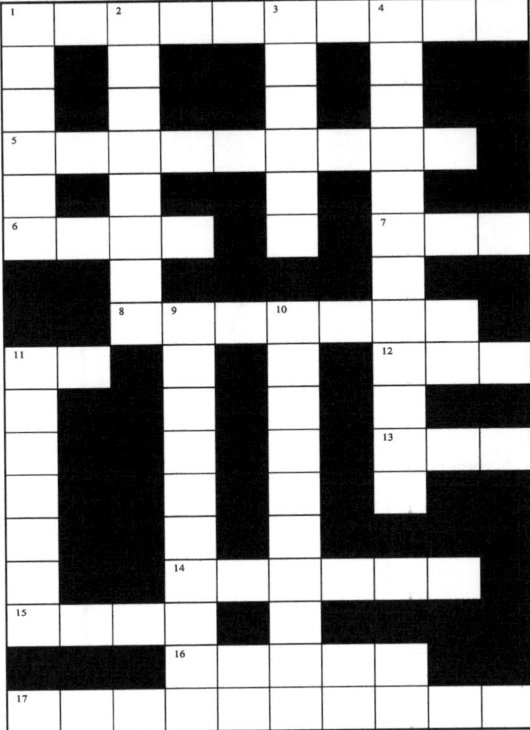

Clues

Across

1.   A chronic neurological disorder that affects the brain's ability to control sleep-wake cycles. (10 letters)

5. Inflammation of the lining of the small, air-filled cavities behind your cheekbones and forehead. (9 letters)

6. Prefix generally meaning "against" or "counter-acting" (4 letters)

7. Medical abbreviation for a severe head injury. (3 letters)

8. An anti-inflammatory medicine. (7 letters)

11. Abbreviation for a well-known bacterial infection, usually in the lungs. (2 letters)

12. An abbreviation for a life-saving technique used in medical emergencies, such as a heart attack. (3 letters)

13. Abbreviation for when a patient chooses to leave the hospital before the treating physician recommends discharge. (3 letters)

14. Existing in hidden or dormant form. (6 letters)

15. Information, facts or statistics. (4 letters)

16. Relating to the nose. (5 letters)

17. Relating to body structure. (10 letters)

Down

1.   A feeling of queasiness such as from motion sickness. (6 letters)
2.   Can be a symptom of allergies. (8 letters)
3.   Medical term for wound, abscess or ulcer. (6 letters)
4.   (*American*) A medical practitioner specializing in children aged 2 to 12 years old. (12 letters)
9. An operation in which an organ or tissue is implanted into a body. (10 letters)
10. An autoimmune disease that can affect joints, tendons, muscles, ligaments and bones. (10 letters)
11. Small, butterfly-shaped gland located at the front of the neck. (7 letters)

Fill in blanks

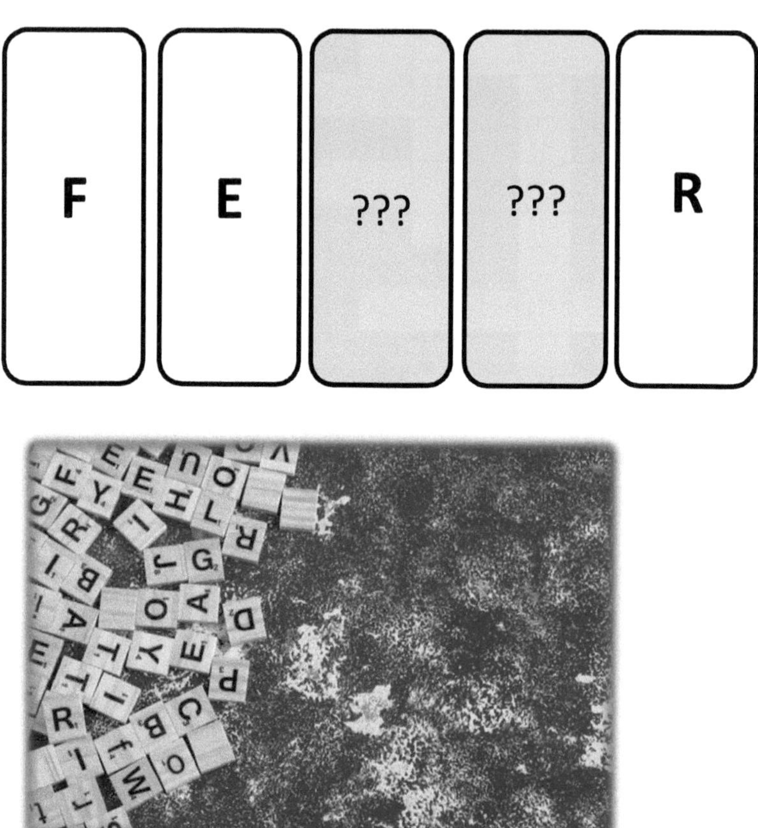

1

Fill in the medical terminology according to the description

a. A   : Disturbance in the electrical activity of the brain

a. B:Surgical Repair of a nerve

a. C:Paralysis on one side of the body

a. D   : Abnormal mental state characterized by confusion, disorientation, and agitation

a. E: The medical term for fainting

a. F: The medical term for an abnormal sensation such as burning or tingling

a. G   : The medical term for an abnormal sensation such as burning or tingling

a. H   : Pathological conditions occurs when there is an accumulation of cerebrospinal fluid in the ventricles of the brain

a. I Diagnostic procedures used to obtain cerebrospinal fluid for analysis

a. J :Medical term meaning pertaining to the ear

a. K   :Medical term meaning double vision

a. L:Normal loss of hearing due to aging

a. M   Tinnitus:Term referring to ringing in the ears

a. N   :Term meaning dizziness.

a. O   :Pathological condition due to an opaque or cloudly lense

a. P :Pathology condition is due to increased intraocular pressure

a. Q   :Pathological condition commonly known as pink eye

a. RSurgical repair of the eyelid.

a. S :Procedure that measures intraocular pressure

a. T:Procedure that examines the auditory canal

a. U   :Term meaning record of hearing

a. V   :X-ray involving injecting dye into the bladder

Multiple choices

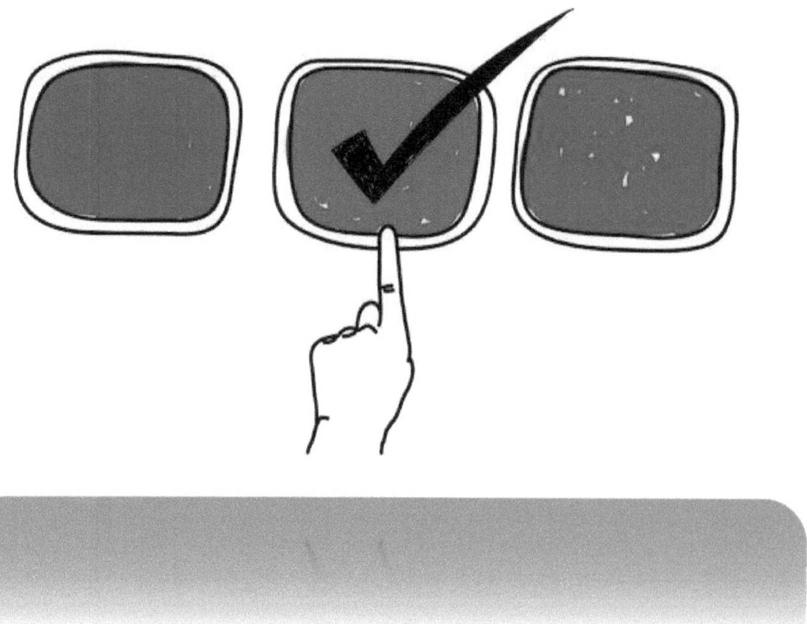

1

- Medical Abbreviations Quiz

1 A blood test used to diagnose and monitor diabetes which indicates blood sugar levels over the past three months
   a. FBS
   b. HbA1c
   c. HGB

2 Abbreviation for a sudden deficient supply of blood to the brain lasting for a short time
   a. CVA
   b. TIA
   c. ALS

Transient ischemic attack (TIA) is like a stroke, but is not a stroke since no permanent damage occurs. CVA is the abbreviation for cerebral vascular accident or stroke.

3 A noninvasive surgical procedure performed to crush kidney or urethral stones

   a. ERCP
   b. ESRD
   c. ESWL

Extracorporeal shock wave lithotripsy (ESWL) uses repeated shockwaves to crush stones in the urinary tract.

4 A test to measure renal function
   a. UA
   b. BUN
   c. KUB

Blood urea nitrogen (BUN) measures the amount of urea in the blood. It is a screening test and an increase may indicate abnormal renal function and /or the need for further study.

Note: BUN is spoken as B-U-N and not bun.

5 Infection of the bladder, ureter and kidney

   a. URI
   b. UTA
   c. UTI

6 The transferring of cells from one body organ to more than one other body organ as in malignant cancer
   a. Ca
   b. met
   c. mets

Metastases (mets) is the plural of metastasis (met).

7 BPH is a condition of the
   a. prostate gland
   b. glans penis
   c. Bartholins gland

Benign prostatic hypertrophy (BPH) is the enlargement of the prostate gland.

8   Identification of the nature of a disease or illness
      a. Dx
      b. Px
      c. Rx

9   A condition that leads to absence of sleep because of repetitive pharyngeal collapse
      a. VPS
      b. OSA
      c. PSG

10   A test to determine levels of carbon dioxide, oxygen, and acidity levels in the blood flowing away from the heart
      a. ABF
      b. CBC
      c. ABG

2

- Medical Terminology Quiz: Blood Clots

1   Phlebitis is inflammation of a (an)

    a.   Vein
    b.   artery
    c.   capillary

Phleb is the word root for vein; phlebitis means inflammation of a vein.

2   Thrombophlebitis means inflammation of a vein due to a(n)

    a.   infection
    b.   plaque
    c.   clot

Thromb is the word root for clot, therefore adding it to the term phlebitis changes the meaning from inflammation of a vein to inflammation of the vein due to a (blood) clot. A blood clot that forms inside of veins or arteries is called athrombus.

3   DVT means:

    a.   deep vein thrombitis
    b.   deep vein thrombosis
    c.   deep vein thrombus

-osis means abnormal condition, therefore thrombosis means abnormal condition of a clot. **Deep vein thrombosis** affects the larger blood vessels, usually deep in the legs in which a piece may break off and travel to the lungs. A **coronary thrombosis** occurs in the arteries that supply the heart, and **cerebral thrombosis** occurs in an artery within the brain.

4   When a small piece of thrombus breaks off and travels through a vessel until it blocks the flow of blood, it is called a(an)

    a.   thrombus
    b.   bruit
    c.   embolus

An **embolus** is a traveling thrombus. (an embolus can also be any material that enters or originates from the vascular system such as air, fat, or bits of any tissue.) The medical condition resulting from an embolus is called an **embolism**. Plural of **embolus** is **emboli**.

5   A noninvasive diagnostic test used to diagnose deep vein thrombosis (DVT) is called

    a.   Doppler ultrasound
    b.   digital subtraction
    c.   sestambi test

A Doppler ultrasound test uses reflected sound waves to see how blood flows through a blood vessel. It helps doctors assess the blood flow through major arteries and veins.

6   Deep vein thrombosis (DVT) is usually a precursor to a thrombus traveling and becoming lodged in a vessel blocking off blood supply to the lung or

    a.   pulmonary embolism

b. pulmonary edema
c. pulmonary neoplasm

PE (pulmonary embolism) can be extremely life threatening since a blocked vessel leading to the lung can impede the exchange of oxygen and carbon dioxide. **A coronary embolism** occurs in the arteries that supply the heart, and **cerebral embolism** occurs in an artery within the brain.

7. Which of the following terms describes complete blockage of a vessel

    a. lumen
    b. occlusion
    c. thrombosis

Occlusion means obstruction or blockage.

8. To diagnose a pulmonary embolism (PE), a series of sectional images using ionizing radiation may be used or

    a. CXR
    b. Chest MRI
    c. Chest CT

CT (computed tomography) produces sectional images of body organs.

9. Thrombolysis means

    a. movement of a clot
    b. formation of a clot
    c. dissolution of a clot

Thrombolysis (**-lysis** means dissolusion), also known as **thrombolytic therapy**, is a treatment to dissolve dangerous clots in blood vessels.

10. Anticoagulants (blood thinners) are often ordered following a PE. The blood test to monitor this therapy is

    a. PT
    b. PP
    c. PE

Prothrombin time (PT) is a blood test that measures how long it takes blood to clot. PT is used to check whether medicine to prevent blood clots is working. A PT test may also be called an INR test.

1) If I haven't been brushing my teeth often enough, I may end up with bleeding from my gums, a condition called

   a. hepatitis

   b. colitis

   c. gingivitis

   d. stomatitis

   e. proctitis

2) A patient has had a diagnosis of colon cancer and will need surgical removal of the colon. She will end up with a permanent hole in her abdomen for drainage into a bag. The permanent opening is called a

   a. megacolon

   b. colitis

   c. colonoscopy

   d. colostomy

   e. colectomy

3) You have been having chronic pains in your upper abdomen, and your family physician refers you to a specialist in diseases of the digestive tract called a

   a. cardiologist

   b. pulmonologist

   c. neurologist

   d. gastroenterologist

   e. proctologist

4) You have just been diagnosed as having an enlarged liver. The doctor describes it as

   a. megacolon

   b. hepatomegaly

   c. macrostomia

   d. hepatitis

   e. gastroenteritis

5) You have taken your friend to the emergency room with severe lower back pain and blood in his urine. After examination and lab tests, the physician reports that your friend has an inflammation of his kidneys and makes a diagnosis of

   a. hepatitis

b. cystitis

c. proctitis

d. nephritis

e. orchiditis

6) Your friend who is a long distance runner is told by his physician that he has an enlarged heart, but that this can be a normal finding in well conditioned athletes. The doctor writes on his chart that your friend has

a. hepatomegaly

b. cardiomegaly

c. megacolon

d. macrostomia

e. myocarditis

7) Your mother is having her uterus surgically removed along with her ovaries. Removal of ovaries is called

a. hysterectomy

b. orchidectomy

c. appendectomy

d. oophorectomy

e. gastrectomy

8) A patient has become sterile due to chronic inflammation of her uterine tubes from frequent infection with sexually transmitted diseases. This tubal inflammation is called

a. endometritis

b. perimetritis

c. salpingitis

d. hepatitis

e. proctitis

9) A patient with epilepsy has had a procedure performed that records brain electrical activity. This procedure is called

a. electrocardiography

b. electroencephalography

c. electromyography

d. electrogastrography

e. electrophoresis

10) A female patient has a special X-ray procedure of the breasts performed. The X-ray image is called a

a. mammoplasty

b. mammoplasia

c. mammography

d. mastectomy

e. mammogram

Who am I?

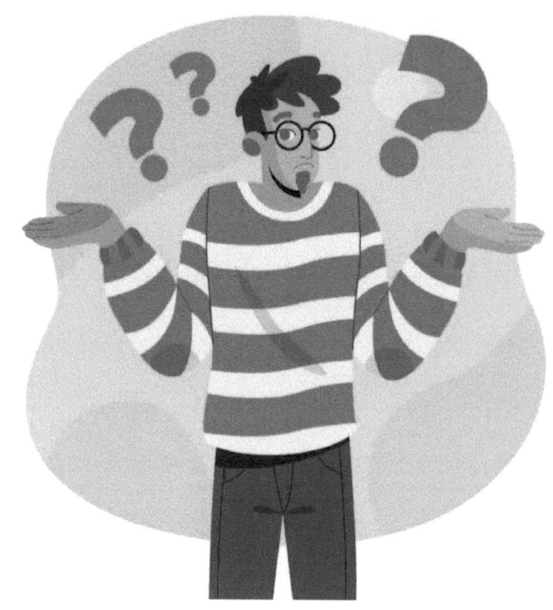

1

- **Organs in (pictures)**

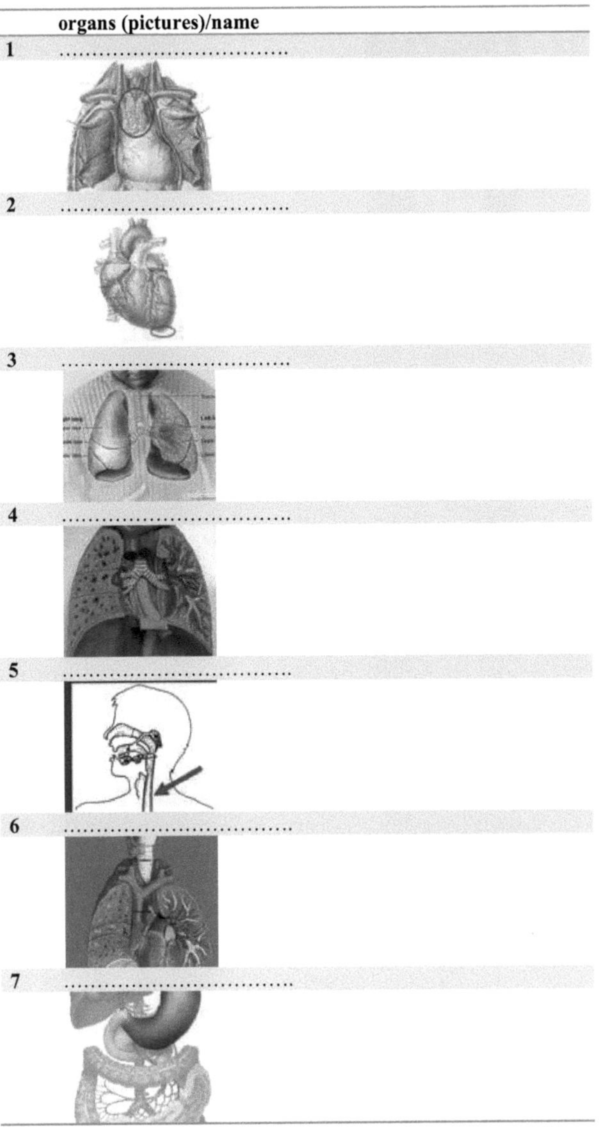

organs (pictures)/name
1 ....
2 ....
3 ....
4 ....
5 ....
6 ....
7 ....

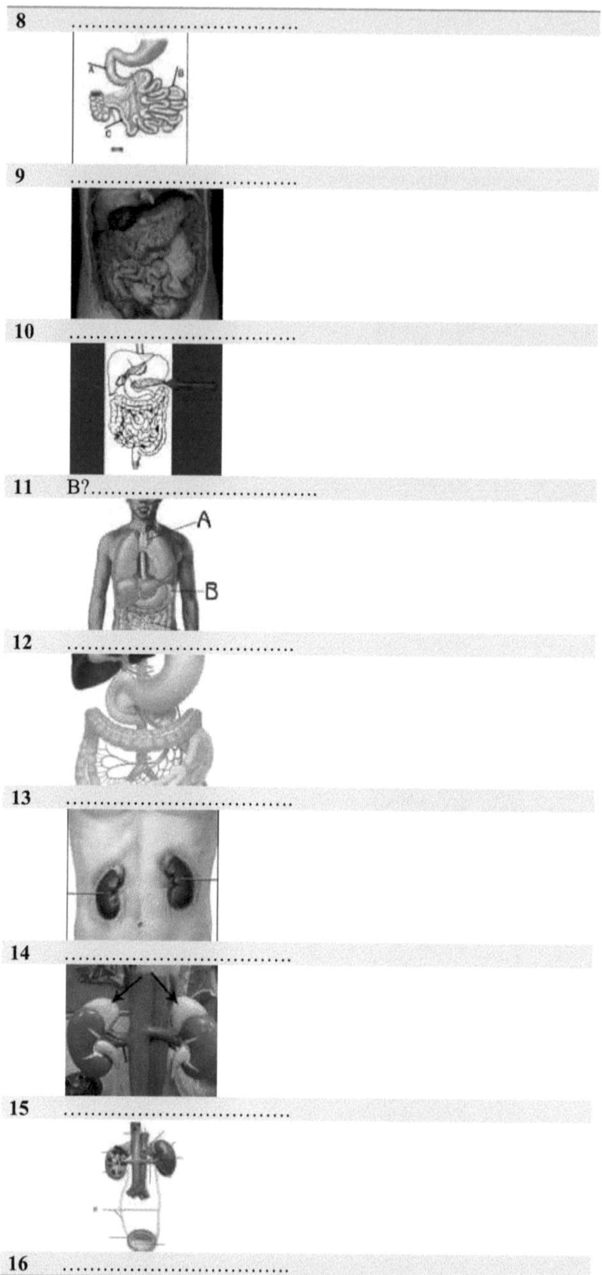

8 ....

9 ....

10 ....

11 B? ....

12 ....

13 ....

14 ....

15 ....

16 ....

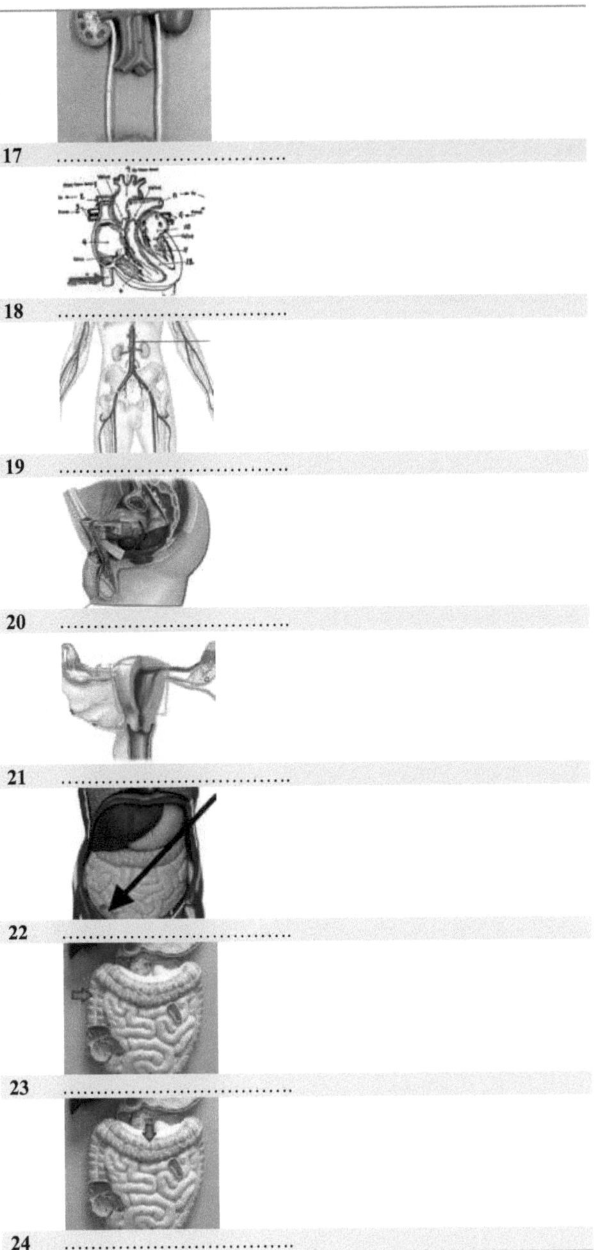

17 ....

18 ....

19 ....

20 ....

21 ....

22 ....

23 ....

24 ....

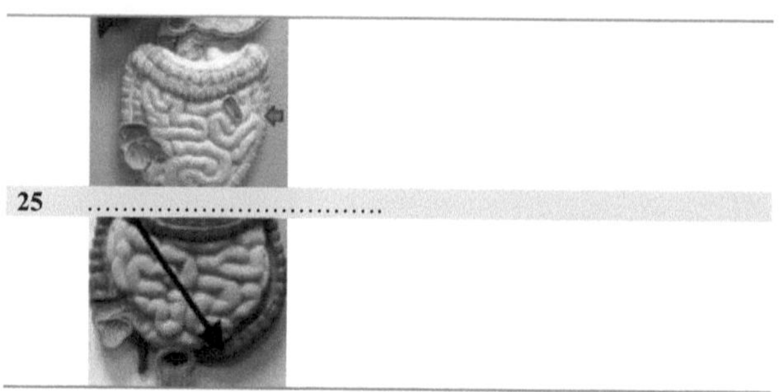

25 ....

2

- **Who am I?**

- **Organ function table**

Organ	Function
....	.... is a worm-like structure attached to the first part of the colon. It has no known function. It can get inflamed and cause pain (appendicitis). We don't miss our appendix if it is removed.
....	.... is where we do our thinking. It also controls body functions that we don't think very hard about such as breathing and walking. The brain stores our memories and controls the nervous system. Diseases of the brain include brain tumours (that can be cancerous or non-cancerous), degenerative brain disease like Huntington's and bacterial infections like meningitis.
....	..............., also known as the large intestine, is the final part of the digestive tract. It packages any food waste and removes water to form solid poo (faeces). If your large intestine gets infected with by harmful bacteria, this can stop it removing waste water and lead to diarrhea. The colon is also the place where bowel cancer can develop.
....	.... pumps blood around our body through a system of arteries. Blood picks up oxygen in the lungs and delivers it to where it is needed. Veins return the deoxygenated blood to the heart. Heart disease is a common cause of poor health and death in the UK. It is most often caused when blood vessels become blocked, leading to heart attack. Many forms of heart disease can be prevented or treated with healthy lifestyle choices.
....	.... are involved in homeostasis, which means regulating the internal environment to keep conditions in the body stable. It does this by regulating excretion of water and other substances. Kidneys can be damaged if they are infected by bacteria, or if a blockage is caused by a build-up of insoluble calcium (kidney stones). Other problems that can occur with kidneys includes the growth of cysts, or damage caused by high blood pressure.
....	.... has many functions including converting nutrients from the diet into a form that the body can use for energy and growth. The liver also breaks down drugs such as alcohol and Paracetamol. There are lots of different types of liver disease including those caused by excessive alcohol consumption, and viral conditions like hepatitis.
....	.... are the organs responsible for taking in oxygen from the air. The oxygen is transferred to the blood so that it can reach every cell in the body. Smoking seriously damages the lungs. Another common cause of lung disease is bacterial infection.
....	.... secretes the hormone insulin, which controls levels of sugar in the blood. It also secretes enzymes that help digest food in the small intestine. Pancreatitis is a condition caused by inflammation of the pancreas, usually caused by stones in the gall bladder.

....	This is the part of the digestive tract between the stomach and the colon. It is where food is digested and nutrients absorbed. The small intestine is about 5 metres long. Problems with the small intestine can include Chron's Disease and Irritable Bowel Syndrom.
....	.... sits under your rib cage on the left and is involved in the filtration of blood to remove any dead cells and infective organisms. It is possible to live without a spleen.
....	.... stores food that is swallowed, secretes enzymes to start digestion, produces acid to kill any infective organisms and contracts to break food into smaller pieces. Stomach diseases include gastritis, stomach cancer and stomach ulcers.
....	Men have two .... (the plural of testis). This is where sperm are made. The testes sit in the scrotum, which hangs outside the body to keep the testes cool. Testicular cancer can usually be treated if detected early.
....	.... are a pair of organs at the back of the throat that help protect against infection. They can become enlarged and inflamed, resulting in painful tonsillitis.
....	The trachea is the tube that links the back of the throat with the lungs. Air that is breathed in travels down the trachea. The trachea is held open by rings of hard cartilage.
....	.... or .... is where babies grow. Eggs are produced in the ovaries and pass down the Fallopian tubes to reach the uterus. Fertilised eggs implant in the wall of the uterus and grow there. Problems with the uterus can include cervical and uterine cancer and fibroids (growths of muscle or other tissue in the uterus).
....	the part of the alimentary canal that connects the throat to the stomach; the gullet. In humans and other vertebrates it is a muscular tube lined with mucous membrane.

Answer key

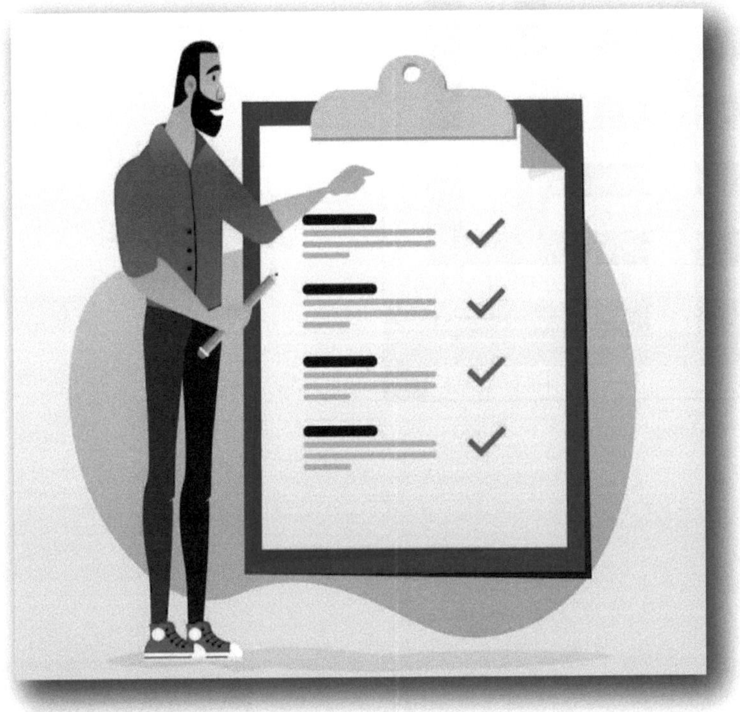

- Crossword puzzle no.1

1	2	3	4	5	6	7	8	9	10	11
¹C	O	N	²G	E	N	I	T	³A	L	■
A	■	■	6	■	■	■	■	⁴P	M	⁵S
⁶R	R	A	P	H	Y	■	■	P	■	P
D	■	■	D	■	■	⁷O	■	E	■	O
I	■	■	■	■	■	B	■	N	■	N
⁸A	B	S	E	N	C	E	■	D	■	D
C	■	■	■	■	■	S	■	E	■	I
■	⁹I	L	L	■	¹⁰Z	I	N	C	■	L
¹¹R	■	■	■	¹²A	■	T	■	T	■	O
¹³A	T	R	O	P	H	Y	■	¹⁴O	I	L
D	■	■	■	L	■	■	■	M	■	Y
¹⁵I	M	¹⁶P	L	A	N	T	■	Y	■	S
A	■	O	■	S	■	■	■	■	■	I
¹⁷T	O	N	S	I	L	L	I	T	I	S
I	■	S	■	A	■	■	■	■	■	■
O	■	■	■	■	■	■	■	■	■	■
¹⁸N	E	U	R	O	P	A	T	H	Y	■

¹N	A	²R	C	O	³L	E	⁴P	S	Y
A		H			E		E		
U		I			S		D		
⁵S	I	N	U	S	I	T	I	S	
E		I			O		A		
⁶A	N	T	I		N		⁷T	B	I
		I					R		
		⁸S	⁹T	E	¹⁰R	O	I	D	
¹¹T	B		R		H		¹²C	P	R
H			A		E		I		
Y			N		U		¹³A	M	A
R			S		M		N		
O			P		A				
I			¹⁴L	A	T	E	N	T	
¹⁵D	A	T	A		I				
			¹⁶N	A	S	A	L		
¹⁷A	N	A	T	O	M	I	C	A	L

- **Fill in blanks**

1

A. Epilepsy: Disturbance in the electrical activity of the brain

| | | | e | P | i | l | e | p | s | y | | |

B. Neuroplasty: Surgical Repair of a nerve

| | | | n | e | U | r | o | p | l | a | s | t | y | |

C. Hemiplegia: Paralysis on one side of the body

| | | | h | e | M | i | p | l | e | g | i | a | |

D. Delirium: Abnormal mental state characterized by confusion, disorientation, and agitation

| | | | d | e | L | i | r | i | u | m | | |

E. Syncope: The medical term for fainting

| | | | s | Y | n | c | o | p | e | | |

F. Paresthesia: The medical term for an abnormal sensation such as burning or tingling

| | | | p | a | R | e | s | t | h | e | s | i | A | |

G. Dementia: The medical term for an abnormal sensation such as burning or tingling

| | | | d | E | m | e | n | t | i | a | | |

H. Hydrocephalus: Pathological conditions occurs when there is an accumulation of cerebrospinal fluid in the ventricles of the brain

| | | | h | Y | d | r | o | c | e | p | h | A | l | u | s |

I. Lumbar Puncture: Diagnostic procedures used to obtain cerebrospinal fluid for analysis

| | | L | u | m | B | a | r | | p | u | n | c | t | u | r | e |

J. Otic: Medical term meaning pertaining to the ear

| | | | | o | t | i | c | | | |

K. Diplopia: Medical term meaning double vision

d	I	p	l	o	p	i	a

L. Presbycusis: Normal loss of hearing due to aging

p	r	e	s	b	y	c	u	s	i	s

M. Tinnitus: Term referring to ringing in the ears

t	i	n	n	i	t	u	s

N. Vertigo: Term meaning dizziness.

v	e	r	t	i	g	o

O. Cataract: Pathological condition due to an opaque or cloudly lense

p	a	t	h	o	l	o	g	i	c	a	l

P. Glaucoma: Pathology condition is due to increased intraocular pressure

G	l	a	u	c	o	m	a

Q. Conjunctivitis: Pathological condition commonly known as pink eye

C	O	n	j	u	n	c	t	i	V	i	t	i	s

R. Blepharoplasty: Surgical repair of the eyelid.

B	L	e	p	h	a	r	o	p	l	a	s	t	Y

S. Tonometry: Procedure that measures intraocular pressure

t	o	n	o	m	e	t	r	r	y

T. Otoscopy: Procedure that examines the auditory canal

o	t	o	s	c	o	p	y

U. Audiogram: Term meaning record of hearing

A	u	d	i	o	g	r	a	m

V. Cystography: X-ray involving injecting dye into the bladder

c	y	s	t	o	g	r	a	p	h	y

- **Multiple choice questions**

1

1	b. HbA1c
2	b. TIA
3	c. ESWL
4	b. BUN
5	c.UTI
6	c.METS
7	a.prostate gland
8	a.Dx
9	b.OSA
10	c.ABG

2

1	Vein
2	Clot
3	Deep vein thrombosis
4	Embolus
5	Doppler ultrasound
6	Pulmonary embolism
7	Occlusion
8	Chest CT
9	Dissolution of a clot
10	prothrombin time (PT)

3

1	Gingivitis
2	Colostomy
3	Gastroenterologist
4	Heptamegaly
5	Nephritis
6	Cardiomegaly
7	Oophorectomy
8	Salpingitis
9	Electroencephalography
10	Mammography

- **Who am I?**

Organs in (pictures)

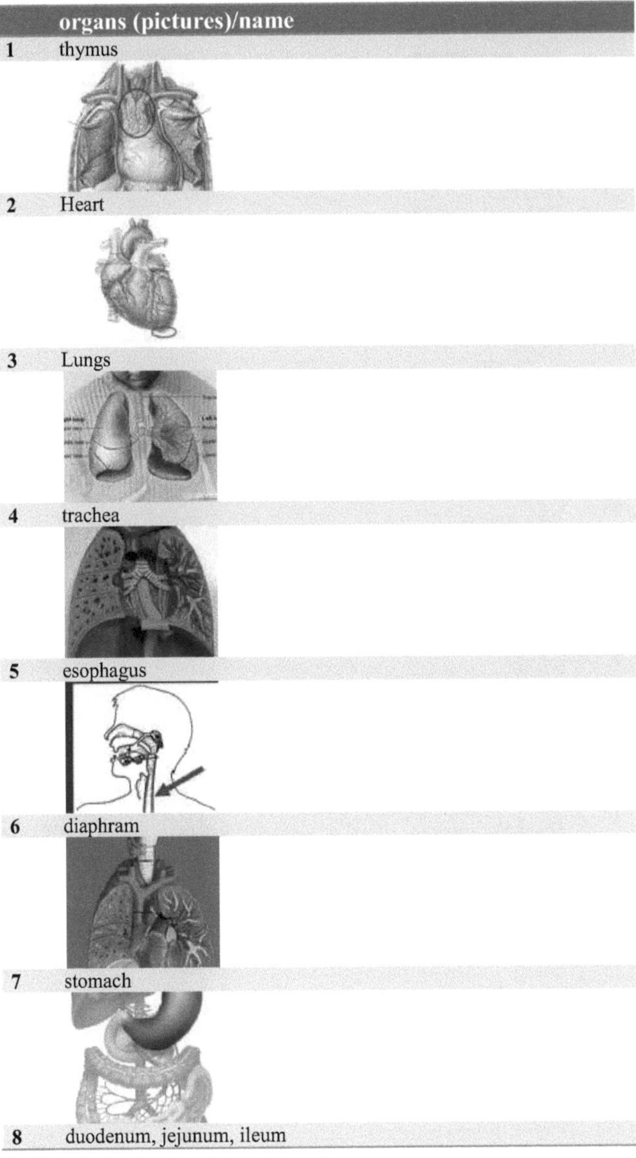

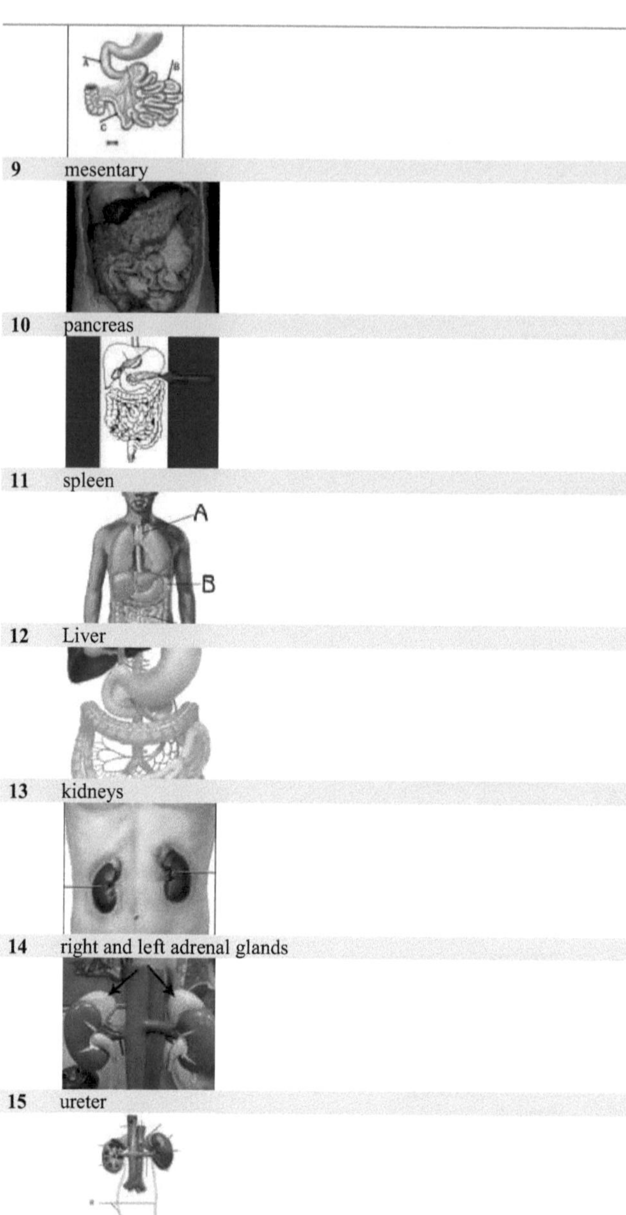

9	mesentary
10	pancreas
11	spleen
12	Liver
13	kidneys
14	right and left adrenal glands
15	ureter
16	urinary bladder

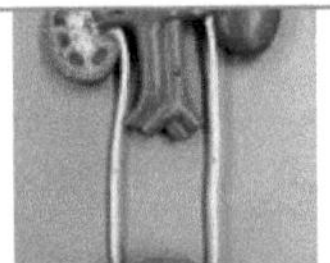

17 inferior vena cava

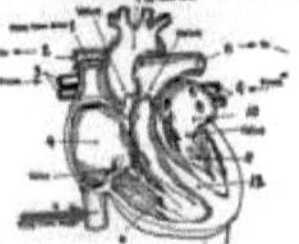

18 abdominal aorta

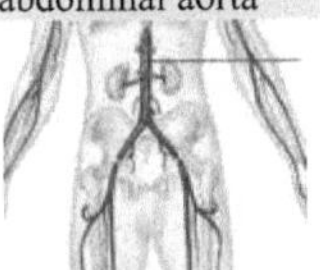

19 testis

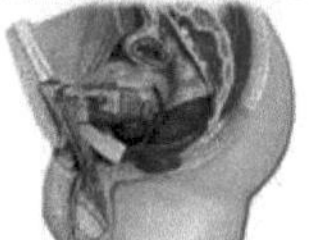

20 uterus

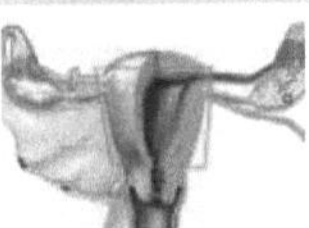

21 cecum

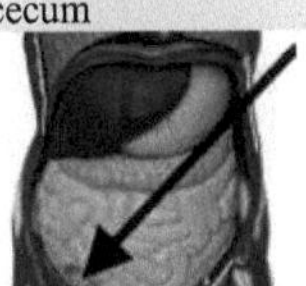

22 ascending colon

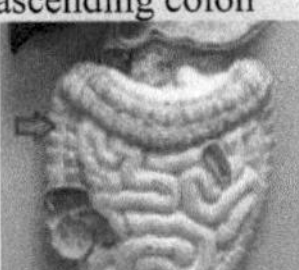

23 transverse colon

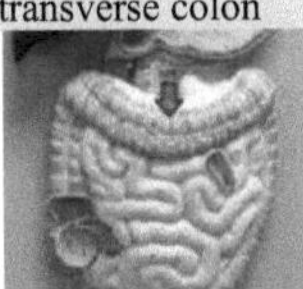

24 descending colon

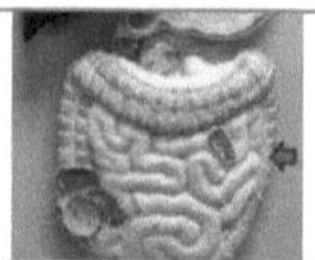
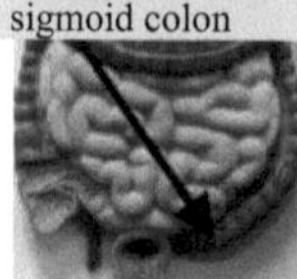

- Organ function table

Organ	Function
Appendix	The appendix is a worm-like structure attached to the first part of the colon. It has no known function. It can get inflamed and cause pain (appendicitis). We don't miss our appendix if it is removed.
Brain	The brain is where we do our thinking. It also controls body functions that we don't think very hard about such as breathing and walking. The brain stores our memories and controls the nervous system. Diseases of the brain include brain tumours (that can be cancerous or non-cancerous), degenerative brain disease like Huntington's and bacterial infections like meningitis.
Colon	The colon, also known as the large intestine, is the final part of the digestive tract. It packages any food waste and removes water to form solid poo (faeces). If your large intestine gets infected with by harmful bacteria, this can stop it removing waste water and lead to diarrhea. The colon is also the place where bowel cancer can develop.
Heart	The heart pumps blood around our body through a system of arteries. Blood picks up oxygen in the lungs and delivers it to where it is needed. Veins return the deoxygenated blood to the heart. Heart disease is a common cause of poor health and death in the UK. It is most often caused when blood vessels become blocked, leading to heart attack. Many forms of heart disease can be prevented or treated with healthy lifestyle choices.
Kidney	The kidneys are involved in homeostasis, which means regulating the internal environment to keep conditions in the body stable. It does this by regulating excretion of water and other substances. Kidneys can be damaged if they are infected by bacteria, or if a blockage is caused by a build-up of insoluble calcium (kidney stones). Other problems that can occur with kidneys includes the growth of cysts, or damage caused by high blood pressure.
Liver	The liver has many functions including converting nutrients from the diet into a form that the body can use for energy and growth. The liver also breaks down drugs such as alcohol and Paracetamol. There are lots of different types of liver disease including those caused by excessive alcohol consumption, and viral conditions like hepatitis.
Lungs	The lungs are the organs responsible for taking in oxygen from the air. The oxygen is transferred to the blood so that it can reach every cell in the body. Smoking seriously damages the lungs. Another common cause of lung disease is bacterial infection.
Pancreas	The pancreas secretes the hormone insulin, which controls levels of sugar in the blood. It also secretes enzymes that help digest food in the small intestine. Pancreatitis is a condition caused by inflammation of the pancreas, usually caused by stones in the gall bladder.
Small Intestine	This is the part of the digestive tract between the stomach and the colon. It is where food is digested and nutrients absorbed. The small intestine is about 5 metres long. Problems with the small intestine can include Chron's Disease and Irritable Bowel Syndrom.
Spleen	The spleen sits under your rib cage on the left and is involved in the filtration of blood to remove any dead cells and infective organisms. It is possible to live without a spleen.

Stomach	The stomach stores food that is swallowed, secretes enzymes to start digestion, produces acid to kill any infective organisms and contracts to break food into smaller pieces. Stomach diseases include gastritis, stomach cancer and stomach ulcers.
Testis	Men have two testes (the plural of testis). This is where sperm are made. The testes sit in the scrotum, which hangs outside the body to keep the testes cool. Testicular cancer can usually be treated if detected early.
Tonsils	The tonsils are a pair of organs at the back of the throat that help protect against infection. They can become enlarged and inflamed, resulting in painful tonsillitis.
Trachea	The trachea is the tube that links the back of the throat with the lungs. Air that is breathed in travels down the trachea. The trachea is held open by rings of hard cartilage.
Uterus	The uterus or womb is where babies grow. Eggs are produced in the ovaries and pass down the Fallopian tubes to reach the uterus. Fertilised eggs implant in the wall of the uterus and grow there. Problems with the uterus can include cervical and uterine cancer and fibroids (growths of muscle or other tissue in the uterus).
Esophagus	the part of the alimentary canal that connects the throat to the stomach; the gullet. In humans and other vertebrates it is a muscular tube lined with mucous membrane.

- **Add your own medical terminology**

Terminology	Arabic	Comment

Terminology	Arabic	Comment
	250	

Terminology	Arabic	Comment
	251	

Terminology	Arabic	Comment
	252	

Terminology	Arabic	Comment
	253	

Terminology	Arabic	Comment
	254	

Terminology	Arabic	Comment
	255	

Terminology	Arabic	Comment
	256	

Terminology	Arabic	Comment
	257	

Terminology	Arabic	Comment
	258	

- **References**

https://www.webteb.com/

https://www.languageonthemove.com/the-interpreting-profession-in-ancient-egypt/

https://www.npr.org/sections/health-shots/2014/10/27/358055673/in-the-hospital-a-bad-translation-can-destroy-a-life

https://www.ncbi.nlm.nih.gov/books/NBK500019/

https://www.lung.org/lung-health-diseases/lung-disease-lookup

https://www.webmd.com/

https://www.niddk.nih.gov/health-information/diagnostic-tests/a1c-test

https://quizlet.com/124153941/med-term-ch-15-nervous-flash-cards/

https://www.freepik.com/

- **Feedback**

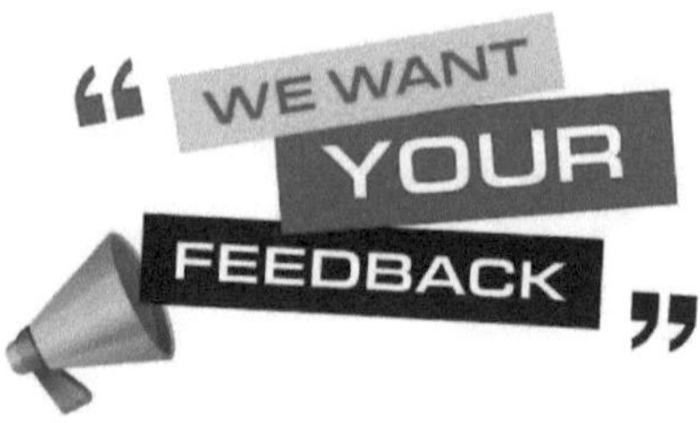

If you enjoyed this book, please take a few moments to write a review of it.

themedicalinterpreterbook@gmail.com

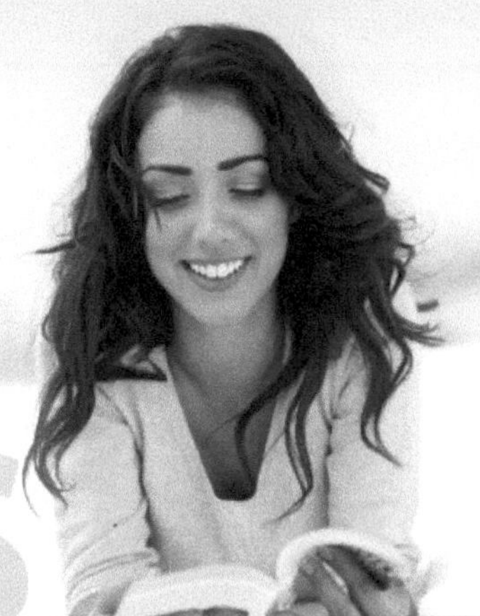

yes
I want morebooks!

Buy your books fast and straightforward online - at one of world's fastest growing online book stores! Environmentally sound due to Print-on-Demand technologies.

Buy your books online at
www.morebooks.shop

Kaufen Sie Ihre Bücher schnell und unkompliziert online – auf einer der am schnellsten wachsenden Buchhandelsplattformen weltweit! Dank Print-On-Demand umwelt- und ressourcenschonend produziert.

Bücher schneller online kaufen
www.morebooks.shop

info@omniscriptum.com
www.omniscriptum.com

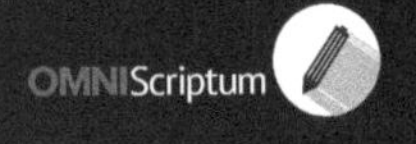